Additional Advance Praise for
EVERY DEEP-DRAWN BREATH

"The ICU is an important, mysterious character in the story of modern medicine, and *Every Deep-Drawn Breath* is its deeply felt, thoroughly researched biography. With compassion, grit, and grace, Dr. Ely takes us into this liminal space and shows us, through the stories of his patients and his life, what it means to mobilize technology to save lives while also confronting the unintended pain and suffering that ICU care can inflict. This book illuminates the humanism, heroism, and humility required to stand with people at life's edge, and reminds us to seek meaning and purpose in the life we have, a life sustained by each breath we take."

—Sunita Puri, MD, author of *That Good Night:*
Life and Medicine in the Eleventh Hour

"In this fascinating and eye-opening book, Wes Ely makes the radical argument that we should be helping critically ill patients stay awake and engaged, not routinely sedating them into unconsciousness. Combining dogged research, intense reflection, and page-turning stories, Dr. Ely reminds us that we have to treat the patient, not just the disease."

—Danielle Ofri, MD, PhD, clinical professor of medicine,
NYU School of Medicine, and author of *When We Do Harm:*
A Doctor Confronts Medical Error

"With the storytelling sensibilities of Oliver Sacks and the surgical precision of Atul Gawande, Dr. Wes Ely has given us an unforgettable journey of patients and doctors traveling in the disorienting world of intensive care, ultimately leading toward redemption for Dr. Ely himself. Required reading for all mortals. If you liked *When Breath Becomes Air*, you will love this book."

—Angelo Volandes, MD, author of *The Conversation:*
A Revolutionary Plan for End-of-Life Care

"*Every Deep-Drawn Breath* is a beautiful, honest gem. If you're interested in the wild world of the ICU, in the interface between nature and human nature, in how medicine (at its best) learns from good intentions gone awry, in the difference between in vitro and in vivo, or in how a good doctor becomes great, here is the book for you. I'm grateful to Dr. Ely for his candor and his storytelling."

—BJ Miller, MD, coauthor of *A Beginner's Guide to the End*

"A remarkable book from a legendary physician. Dr. Ely revolutionized critical care and now, through stories that are intimate, honest, and brave, he reveals the failings and the great promise of the field. This could not be more timely—in the wake of a pandemic that challenged the humanity of our profession, Ely shows us the road forward. A must-read."

—Daniela Lamas, MD, author of *You Can Stop Humming Now: A Doctor's Stories of Life, Death, and in Between*

"*Every Deep-Drawn Breath* is an enthralling journey through the ongoing evolution of critical care. In this richly illustrated book, with stories of people who teetered on the edge of death and survived to find their lives forever changed, Dr. Ely, a thought leader in his field, reveals hard lessons he's learned, innovations he's led, and his compelling, bright vision for the future of medicine."

—Ira Byock, MD, active emeritus professor, Geisel School of Medicine at Dartmouth, author of *Dying Well* and *The Best Care Possible*, and founder and chief medical officer of the Institute for Human Caring

"A stunning, heartbreaking, and hopeful book, expressing Dr. Ely's profound union of compassion and medical skill. Given that most of us will stay in an ICU, attend a loved one there, or even die in one, I hope that many readers demand treatment according to the humane practices Dr. Ely has pioneered. I equally hope that every critical care doctor and hospital administrator reads this beautiful book, puts its protocols into practice, and makes their ICUs more humane and medically effective."

—Katy Butler, author of *Knocking on Heaven's Door* and *The Art of Dying Well*

"A treasure trove of hard-won wisdom. Reading *Every Deep-Drawn Breath* is like getting a backstage pass to the cloistered world of medical science. A gifted storyteller, Wes Ely brings his humanity to every moment, inspiring us to reexamine our own beliefs and reimagine what is possible. He has seamlessly woven together the private stories behind the very public successes and failures of our well-intentioned ICU care. Illuminating and generous, he revisits with humility the pivotal moments of his career in this wise gift of a book."

—Rana Awdish, MD, author of *In Shock: My Journey from Death to Recovery and the Redemptive Power of Hope*

EVERY DEEP-DRAWN BREATH

A Critical Care Doctor on Healing, Recovery, and
Transforming Medicine in the ICU

Wes Ely, MD

SCRIBNER

New York   London   Toronto   Sydney   New Delhi

Scribner
An Imprint of Simon & Schuster, Inc.
1230 Avenue of the Americas
New York, NY 10020

First Scribner hardcover edition September 2021

SCRIBNER and design are registered trademarks of The Gale Group, Inc., used under license by Simon & Schuster, Inc., the publisher of this work.

For information about special discounts for bulk purchases, please contact Simon & Schuster Special Sales at 1-866-506-1949 or business@simonandschuster.com.

The Simon & Schuster Speakers Bureau can bring authors to your live event. For more information or to book an event, contact the Simon & Schuster Speakers Bureau at 1-866-248-3049 or visit our website at www.simonspeakers.com.

Interior design by Wendy Blum

Manufactured in the United States of America

1   3   5   7   9   10   8   6   4   2

Library of Congress Cataloging-in-Publication Data

Names: Ely, E. Wesley, author.
Title: Every deep-drawn breath : a critical care doctor on healing, recovery, and transforming medicine in the ICU / Wes Ely.
Description: First Scribner hardcover edition. | New York : Scribner, 2021. | Includes bibliographical references and index.
Identifiers: LCCN 2021020531 (print) | LCCN 2021020532 (ebook) | ISBN 9781982171148 (hardcover) | ISBN 9781982171179 (ebook)
Subjects: MESH: Critical Care | Intensive Care Units | Treatment Outcome | Critical Illness | Aftercare | Personal Narrative
Classification: LCC RA975.5.I56 (print) | LCC RA975.5.I56 (ebook) | NLM WX 218 | DDC 616.02/8—dc23
LC record available at https://lccn.loc.gov/2021020531
LC ebook record available at https://lccn.loc.gov/2021020532

ISBN 978-1-9821-7114-8
ISBN 978-1-9821-7117-9 (ebook)

To Kim, for your Love

To Mom, for your English

To Dad, for your Engineering

To Taylor, Blair, and Brooke, for your Understanding

And to the pickers, patients, and others, who continue to teach me what matters

Sometimes a kind of glory lights up the mind of a man. It happens to nearly everyone. You can feel it growing or preparing like a fuse burning toward dynamite. It is a feeling in the stomach, a delight of the nerves, of the forearms. The skin tastes the air, and every deep-drawn breath is sweet. Its beginning has the pleasure of a great stretching yawn; it flashes in the brain and the whole world glows outside your eyes.

—John Steinbeck, *East of Eden*

Contents

Author's Note   xi

Prologue   1

Chapter 1:   13
Fractured Lives—Embracing a New Normal

Chapter 2:   27
Early History of Critical Care—Bumpy Gravel Roads to
ICU Interstates

Chapter 3:   45
Culture of Critical Care—The Era of Deep Sedation and
Immobilization

Chapter 4:   57
The World of Transplant Medicine—Harvesting the
Right Path Forward

Chapter 5:   75
Delirium Disaster—An Invisible Calamity for Patients
and Families

Chapter 6:   95
The View from the Other Side of the Bed—
Illness Revisited

Contents

Chapter 7:   103
Deciding My Path—Combining Research with
Clinical Care

Chapter 8:   115
Unshackling the Brain—Finding Consciousness in the
ICU

Chapter 9:   133
Awakening Change—Patients Are Resurfacing

Chapter 10:   155
Spreading the Word—Putting New Ideas into Practice

Chapter 11:   179
Finding the Person in the Patient—Hope through
Humanization

Chapter 12:   209
End-of-Life Care in the ICU—Patient and Family Wishes
Can Come True

Epilogue   233

Resources for Patients, Families, Caregivers,
    and Medical Professionals   247
Books to Explore   276
Acknowledgments   279
Notes   283
Index   313

Author's Note

MANY PEOPLE BELIEVE MEDICINE is grounded in benevolence, that is, *wishing* good. It is more than that. The target principle of medicine must be a higher standard: beneficence. *Doing* good. This breeds trust between my patient and me, which is the cornerstone of my art and practice. In return for her trust, I promise always to try to help her, and never harm her. Every time I step into the hospital, I remind myself of the enormity of this promise. This covenant.

Early in my career, I strayed. Not intentionally, but out of a desire to control every medical circumstance, I didn't listen well enough. Our greatest treasure is found in deep, real communication with each other. When this is nurtured, especially in times of suffering, two people can establish something of almost mystical quality: a reciprocal connection that brings us to a place of charity and empathy that crosses cultural, social, and racial boundaries. Without such communication, we remain miles apart.

As a young ICU doctor, I went to extreme lengths in my sole focus on saving lives. In so doing, I sometimes sacrificed patient dignity and caused harm. This happened when I traded the priceless gift of eye contact and conversation for medically induced unconsciousness and many hundreds of hours of deep sedation that I thought were "required." One by one, patients and their loved ones began to reveal to me the error in my thinking. I had broken our covenant by taking away the patient's voice in his own medical narrative, which is to say, in his life. The journey back to my original oath—first do no harm—brought me to write this book.

The good news is that I—we—now know better. As a physician

and a scientist, working with teams of colleagues, I have helped create a better way forward that brings healing. Lessons I learned through the individual bedside experiences brought to life in this book proved true on a larger scale, as many thousands of patients consented for us to use their time, illness, and blood as part of international investigations. In a real sense, this is their story. Their lives also endowed me with truths that apply well beyond medicine and into every moment of my life.

Nearly everyone will either be an ICU patient or someday worry desperately about a loved one experiencing life-threatening illness. This became excruciatingly clear during the COVID-19 pandemic, when the intense isolation of our approach to infection with the coronavirus rendered millions of people alone and depersonalized. Indeed, one of my hopes is that the enduring lessons we learn from patients in this book, and subsequent improvements in our approach as healers, will be utilized now and for decades to come as tools in a future pandemic. No one chooses to be a patient, but everyone can choose to keep sight of the person in the hospital gown. Each patient is more than a mere beating heart or breathing lungs to be saved. The whole person—mind, body, and spirit—is at stake.

My "why" in medicine is about finding the person in the patient, using touch first and technology second. The powerful combination of humanity and compassion, enmeshed within our modern technological world, is the best way to do good for others. It is the vow I keep, going forward as a physician, and it is how I will do better, more broadly, as a husband, father, son, brother, and friend.

E. Wesley Ely, MD, MPH

THIS IS A BOOK of narrative nonfiction. No made-up stories or dreamed-up scenarios. First and foremost, therefore, I am indebted to the people who agreed to share intimate and highly personal aspects of their life stories with me through recorded interviews. I used real names with written permission except in the following instances: one deceased patient's family asked me to use an alias, though the medical details of her story remain factual. I also used aliases for three Haitian patients and modified details of their stories to protect their identity.

EVERY DEEP-DRAWN BREATH

Prologue

At times life takes on the shape of art, and the remnants
of moments are largely what we come to mean by life . . .
our long certain tragedies, and our springtime lyrics and
limericks make up most of what we are.

—Norman Maclean, *Young Men and Fire*

IT WAS ALMOST SUNRISE and my shift was nearly over, just a young man's leg fracture to set and I'd be done. I stretched and looked up, and there in the trauma bay was Ruthie the Duck Lady, her dirty-white duck quacking from a shoebox, its neck poking through a hole in the worn cardboard top. Ruthie was a local legend, a tourist attraction, and I'd spotted her and her duck many times in the French Quarter, but this was my first time seeing her here in the hospital. Blood dripped down Ruthie's split brow. Thugs had beaten her up and she had, like so many others in New Orleans when a medical issue arose, trekked over to Charity Hospital to see us. I got right to work cleaning her wounds and asking a jillion long-wondered questions as I stitched her up, my voice raised above the honking of the duck.

When we were done, she handed me the duck-in-a-box and danced a frenzied jig of thanks for all of us in the emergency room, her legs flying out like a Cossack's doing the hopak, and I rushed to join in. I'd been doing this dance since my college days, although never before with a duck in my hands. We all laughed together. Only at Charity. There

1

was no thought of paperwork. In my years there, I never saw anyone turned away, regardless of insurance status or financial means. Some payments came to us as canisters of crawfish étouffée, boiled crabs, or Cajun-spiced andouille in Styrofoam coolers. As Ruthie left, the new day's sun slipped through the sliding glass doors and more sick folks streamed in.

I'd come to New Orleans a couple of years earlier as a Tulane medical student in 1985. Charity Hospital, a 250-year-old refuge in the sweaty South, provided health care to the poorest of the poor. Its air was heavy with history. Alton Ochsner, Michael DeBakey, and Rudolph Matas, icons in medicine and surgery, had trained there decades before and left their marks of excellence. For years, Charity had been the largest hospital in the country, and at night we medical students would sneak up to the roof of the central twenty-story tower and peer over the 2,680-bed behemoth, contemplating the great chasm between where we were, and where we needed to be, in becoming physicians. It was a dizzying feeling. All those sick people down there who needed care, who were putting their trust in us. One such night, my roommate Darin Portnoy and I made a pact that we'd steer our medical journeys to help the people who needed us most, the people without a voice. Perhaps the Ruthies of the world.

In the 1980s, Charity functioned mainly on federal and state funds paid to hospitals caring for huge uninsured populations, and its poverty showed. We routinely ran out of bandages and gauze and filed X-rays under patients' mattresses for safekeeping. Without a budget for phlebotomists and patient transport, the med students and doctors-in-training drew all the blood and wheeled patients to their procedures. Some days the power went out, leaving windowless hallways dark and labs shuddering to a halt. We just kept on going. One night, I had to hold a penlight in my mouth to deliver a baby, moving my neck to dart the angle of the beam up to see the mother's face, then the blood pressure monitor, and back down to catch the baby.

The emergency room was always full, packed so tight we'd have to walk in zigzags, back and forth, just to get through the masses of people waiting to be tended. It was both a local clinic and a trauma center, for those with the flu, advanced cancer, gunshot wounds, and everything in between. People screamed in pain, pleading for relief, the constant din a soundtrack to our work, urging us on. The humanity at Charity ran as thick as a slow-cooked, Mississippi River–brown roux. I couldn't get enough of it.

• • •

For the five summers prior to college, I'd worked as a farmhand in huge produce fields just south of my hometown of Shreveport, Louisiana, filling wooden bushel baskets with purple hull peas, Kentucky Wonder green beans, bell peppers, tomatoes, okra, and earthy hand-dug potatoes. Money was scarce for our family. My father had left years earlier to pursue a life apart from us, and my mother's job as an English teacher at a local Jesuit high school didn't bring in much, so the wages I earned under the relentless Southern sun helped out.

The men I worked alongside—Black, brown, and white, formally educated and not, young and old—welcomed me each year. As we talked in the half-light before dawn, tossing hay bales up into the dusty rafters of the old barn, I felt I belonged. But I didn't. As I grew older, I began to see the divide that separated the pickers' lives from mine. The obvious differences at first: that I would move away, out into the world, while they would stay, constantly pouring themselves into the fields but never advancing. This was their entire life, and no matter how hard they toiled or dreamed, change might never come. And then the seemingly smaller things: abscessed teeth that turned into huge gaps in their smiles, a bruised leg that never healed, the cuts and scrapes that didn't get the stitches they needed and so oozed, attracting flies. A minor ailment that they might dismiss for a month or a year or two, laughing it off, until maybe it wasn't so minor. Perhaps it would even prevent them from earning a living. I began to understand that the pickers couldn't afford to stop working long enough to help themselves, even if their lives depended on it. They didn't have the safety net that I did. I saw the ways I was supported by the many people around me who guided me and lifted me up. If I did fall, it wouldn't be too far.

The summer before I started working on the farm, my mother organized a book club for five of my swim team friends and me. We swam twice a day, about fifteen thousand yards before the sun set, reading and discussing the books my mom suggested in between. John Steinbeck's *Of Mice and Men. A Separate Peace* by John Knowles. S. E. Hinton's *The Outsiders*. I was riveted by *I Know Why the Caged Bird Sings* by Maya Angelou, her memoir of growing up in Stamps, Arkansas, and I imagined her up there just to the north. I had never read anything like it before and couldn't stop thinking about the long shadow of trauma and injustice in her life, the heavy weight of her silence. As I worked alongside the pickers, I often thought of the young Maya. Her lack of a voice in her own story paralleled their lives. While I knew she had regained her voice later, in blazing splendor, I feared that wouldn't happen for Marcelo, Marcos, Charlie, and Germain—our mainstay pickers. I had the feeling that even if they were to scream, no one would hear them.

• • •

My desire to become a doctor was sown in those fertile fields, a youthful notion of wanting to help others, and by a quote I held close from *Of Mice and Men.* When George says, "We got a future . . . ," Lenny breaks in with "An' why? Because . . . because I got you to look after me, and you got me to look after you, and that's why." I liked the idea of being there for people who needed me. When I arrived at Charity, I felt I'd truly found my calling.

In my third year of medical school, my first patient was Sarah Bollich. Sarah had grown up in a clapboard shotgun house on Desire

Street in the Ninth Ward in East New Orleans. She was twenty-three years old with a one-week-old baby and should have been at home bonding with her newborn child. Instead, she huddled in a brown blanket in the large open-ward intensive care unit in profound shock. Sarah was sick with peripartum cardiomyopathy, a rare and deadly disease of the heart muscle that occurs in a small number of pregnant or postpartum women. When I first met Sarah, she looked at me, her eyes full of fear, as if she were praying for help but couldn't get the words out. She was terrified she was going to die. We were the same age.

As a student, my job was to watch over her, staying by her paint-chipped metal bed for hours. I examined Sarah using the time-honored sequence of steps: inspection, palpation, percussion, and auscultation. She was straining to breathe, using extra muscles in her neck and chest just to get enough air. Monitoring her blood pressure, I became anxious every time it dipped into the fifties, well below the seventy millimeters of mercury I was told to maintain. We didn't have the new electronic pumps at Charity, so I dialed dopamine by hand, manually counting the drops per minute as the drug flowed from the IV bag through the tubing into Sarah's vein. Too little and her blood pressure would go down. Then I'd increase the number of drops, rolling my finger along the tubing to titrate the dose, trying to bring her pressure back up. It was tedious work, but it meant I spent a good deal of time with Sarah, hoping her heart would get better. Beyond the curtains pulled tight around her bed, the busy world of the ICU pulsed and beeped, all noise and movement. But in here my focus was on her. I held her right hand and she gripped mine, her palm sweaty with fear.

"What's happening to me, Dr. Wes?" she asked again and again. Or "Why can't I be home with my baby?" Unsure of myself and my nascent knowledge, I fumbled through some facts. Her blood pressure was too low. Her heart was failing. We hoped it would improve. We both knew that she was likely to die. I could see it in her eyes, and I'm sure she could see it in mine. But she continued to trust my medicine, and me.

One evening, Sarah's blood pressure plummeted again, way down into the forties. I rolled my finger along the tubing and watched as the drop rate increased. She'd need a lot of fluid and dopamine this time. I turned to reassure her once more and saw stark terror on her face. She grabbed my hand and I froze, holding tight to her fingers. The rhythm on her monitor changed to V-tach, reflecting her dangerously racing heart, and alarms started sounding. I felt her grip loosen. Nurses and residents rushed in to take charge of the code. They slipped a tube down her throat and started CPR, trying to get Sarah's heart rhythm back. Then it was my turn. I'd never given chest compressions before, and I pushed down, released, and down again, my palms hard on her chest, desperate to send blood to her brain to keep her alive. Nothing worked. Her body gave way, and all I could do was stare at the desolate flat line on the monitor. We hadn't been able to fix her heart—we just didn't have the tools.

Perhaps I should have accepted Sarah's death as the inevitable outcome of a terrible disease, but I couldn't. I felt injured. To me, a student doctor, it seemed completely wrong. She'd been so young and healthy, with her whole life ahead of her. She'd grown up watching tankers and paddleboats go down the Mississippi River, wondering where they were heading and if she'd ever travel there, too. Now she wouldn't. She was gone. I couldn't bear the thought of this happening again. I realized that I wanted to do much more than just help people. That idea suddenly seemed pointless, like a teenager's half-baked musings. I wanted to push back against death. That day, I knew that committing myself to critical care medicine, saving lives in extremis, was my vocation. I felt excited about the decision and promised to immerse myself in the best training and the latest technology to save the next Sarah. And all the Sarahs after her.

• • •

In 1989, I had graduated medical school and was a resident-in-training at Wake Forest Medical Center (formerly Bowman Gray). On my first rotation in the ICU, I was assigned to a patient named Teresa Martin. When I first saw Teresa, she was on life support—sedated and paralyzed with medications, and connected to a ventilator by a plastic tube down her throat. The coloring of her arms and legs was off, ashen and mottled at the same time. She'd arrived in the ICU thirty minutes earlier, rushed in by ambulance after a suicide attempt. She'd taken a handful of pills, lost consciousness, and inhaled vomit. Now her lungs, heart, and kidneys were all in different stages of failing. The paramedics had found her sobbing, mumbling she had made a stupid mistake, that she didn't really want to die, before passing out again. She was twenty-eight years old. As an intern training in internal medicine, I vowed to do everything in my power to keep her alive. This time, unlike at Charity, I had an entire arsenal of critical care equipment to help me succeed.

First, Teresa needed a central IV line placed into her heart to measure blood pressure and deliver antibiotics, fluids, and medications. We interns fought to take over this kind of complex procedure so we could learn, and I immediately began prepping her, scrubbing her neck and torso with Betadine, covering her body with a sky-blue sterile drape, and placing a series of needles and dilators through her skin to steer the catheter into the internal jugular vein in her neck and then down into her heart. With that done, I'd bought some time for her body to begin to recover. My job now was to manage her ventilator, IV meds, and sedation, and to check the monitors for signs that her organs were getting better.

Three days later, her kidneys started shutting down—a step in the wrong direction—but I had a fix for it. Another catheter into her groin, more needles, more blood draws, and the beginning of dialysis, filtering her blood using a plastic kidney placed upright, as if standing at attention, a few feet from her head. I paused to look at Teresa, small and alone in her hospital bed, unconscious and surrounded by beeping machines that were keeping her alive. She was a patient without a voice, and I wanted to do my best for her.

Teresa was under my care for weeks and began to look like a pincushion, her skin bruised and oozing from all the blood draws. Her lungs, stiffened by pneumonia, ruptured six times, collapsing over and over, and each time I was able to save her by cutting into her chest and inserting plastic tubes between her ribs. It seemed extraordinary, the number of ways we could push death away.

Throughout this endless cascade of procedures, we kept Teresa deeply sedated with a benzodiazepine drip and gave her morphine for the pain. We did this for all our patients, hoping to spare them the anxiety of being in the ICU, to prevent them from feeling scared. Teresa's parents came by twice a day, their faces pinched and drawn, showing up for the hospital's visiting hours to stare at their unconscious daughter. I didn't have anything concrete to tell them, just that we were doing our best, using the latest technology to save their daughter's life. Her mother was often in tears, standing at the end of Teresa's bed. "I can't understand why she did it. She seemed so happy," her mother said. I never knew what to say.

Finally, Teresa's shock resolved and her blood pressure stabilized. I was able to remove the ventilator. It was as if she were slowly coming back to life, returning to herself, one organ at a time. Her kidneys were still a problem, though, and we carried on with dialysis. The long weeks since her admission dragged on. Her parents were exhausted, silent, not daring to hope anymore, yet not daring not to. Then, gradually, over the next few days, her kidneys started up again. I let out an immense sigh of relief, as if I'd been holding my breath since Teresa arrived. After watching over all those machines, turning dials, and responding to beeps and buzzers, I proudly told her mom and dad that she was going to be okay. That against the odds, she had survived.

• • •

After further recovery in the hospital, Teresa was able to go home. Six weeks later, she came in for a follow-up check on her chest wounds.

I hoped they were healing well. She rolled slowly into the room in a wheelchair, pushed by an aide, her mother at her side. She gazed ahead, heavy bags under her eyes, a shell of a young woman. No greeting, no smile. She turned to me with a blank stare, and I wasn't sure if she remembered me at all.

Almost immediately Teresa's mom asked, "Why can't she bend her arms at the elbows or move her shoulders?" Her mom looked drained, more tired even than when she'd visited her daughter in the hospital. We ran through a litany of other problems that Teresa was having. She couldn't swallow properly or sleep or go to the bathroom alone. She couldn't shower or dress herself. She could walk only a few steps at a time, and stairs were impossible. The idea of returning to her old job as an administrative assistant was exhausting. The list of ailments was dizzying. I had no immediate solutions for any of it, and even less understanding of where the problems were coming from, so I did what I knew how to do: I ordered blood work and X-rays.

The labs didn't show anything alarming, but the X-ray images of her arms and legs revealed large calcium deposits in her elbows, shoulders, and knees. Teresa had heterotopic ossification, a condition in which bone develops where it shouldn't due to extreme inflammation and prolonged immobilization. It was as if she had rocks growing inside her joints. I had never seen anything like it before and didn't know what to think.

Teresa didn't react at all when I showed her the disturbing images, but her mother nodded in affirmation, as if she now had permission to talk about other concerns. She told me that Teresa's brain wasn't working properly, that she would forget things, people's names, that she'd grown afraid. Mrs. Martin stopped and shifted in her seat. "She's a completely different person now." She glanced at her daughter sitting next to her in the wheelchair and sighed.

After Teresa and her mother left, I sat in the room alone, my door closed against the world. Usually when I finished with a patient, I'd ask for the next one right away. Not this time. Earlier that morning, I'd seen the name *Teresa Martin* on my list of scheduled patients and imagined a triumphant reunion. A cheerful "You've given me a whole new lease on life!" At the very least, a smile. I'd thought she would have been back at work by now, laughing with her friends, enjoying life after her close brush with death. Instead, she was a broken young woman in a wheelchair whose life now was much worse than the one she'd lived just a few months ago before coming under my care. What if she never walked again? What if her brain was permanently injured? In my gut I knew that something about the care she had received in the ICU had damaged Teresa. She had come in with failing organs, and we had fixed them, but somehow she had acquired completely different ailments. New trauma to her body and her brain. I thought I'd found my calling, pulling patients back from the maw of death, but now I wasn't so sure. I started to wonder if saving lives was also causing harm.

• • •

My path through the world of modern medicine is the basis for this book. After my treatment of Teresa Martin, I set out to understand how critical care had strayed from its hopeful beginnings and lost its way. How cutting-edge technology could both exponentially improve survival rates for those with critical illness and unintentionally lower the quality of life for many of those survivors. And whether saving lives should be the only goal for ICU doctors. Along the way, I discovered that the loss of humanity that occurred in medicine over the last fifty years is an essential component of this story. It is imperative that we all change the culture of critical care, entrenched as it may be, and modify the way health care is delivered in the ICU. Our patients' lives depend on it. Through their stories, you will experience what it looks like to have your life saved, to be a "good outcome" for doctors, only to return home to a life so limited you might sometimes wish you hadn't survived at all. You'll learn why the classic "sedate and immobilize" standard of ICU care for patients on ventilators should be discarded. And you'll see a remarkable move toward rehumanization in health care that's underway in thousands of ICUs, including my own, where doctors and nurses heal the world's sickest patients with complete care—technology plus touch. This return to humanity, a comprehensive and evidence-based approach, offers hope to critically ill patients and their families. It's time to make it available everywhere.

In the United States alone, the average person will have more than one ICU stay in their lifetime, and more than 6 million patients will land in intensive care each year. One of them might be you—or a loved one— and the care you receive will directly impact your quality of life after you return home. This book will empower you to advocate for better treatment, for care that puts the patient first and focuses on life beyond the ICU. Or perhaps you are a survivor of critical illness—or know someone who is—and you'll recognize yourself in the stories that follow and realize you're not alone, and that there are resources to help you. I hope so.

Clearly, the arc of critical illness does not end when a patient leaves the ICU, but extends far beyond the hospital into the home, family, and community. It is the responsibility of critical care doctors such as myself to follow along. To play a supportive role in this life we have saved. To give each patient a voice, and to listen to what the patient is saying.

Chapter 1

Fractured Lives—Embracing a New Normal

Severe illness wasn't life-altering, it was life-shattering.

—Paul Kalanithi, *When Breath Becomes Air*

BORN IN TENNESSEE IN 1955, Richard Langford was a preacher's son, destined to be a leader and a servant of the downtrodden in then sleepy Nashville. His grandfather started churches across Missouri and Tennessee, and Richard's parents had their own church just off Music Row. There, Richard grew up, learning to speak with confidence and find his way through a life of modest means. Before school in the mornings, he walked door-to-door selling Bozo the Clown cards for a penny each. A few years later, he was elected student body president, and in college he led the university's student council. All of this culminated in his calling to become a third-generation preacher.

But first Richard would get married, have two daughters, and struggle through a difficult divorce. After he earned his doctor of ministry degree, he opened a church on Eighteenth Avenue South in Nashville and served as a pastor. Eventually he took his savings and became a missionary in the Caribbean and Ethiopia, also working for the World Health Organization. He could recite thousands of Bible verses by heart, chapter and verse, interpreting them and weaving them into the meaning of others' struggles in a healing fashion.

"Those were the richest years of my life," he says, nodding, his glasses slightly askew. I've never heard his life story before. I'm here as a friend, checking in on him after a recent abdominal surgery. Richard grins, remembering, leaning back in a beige La-Z-Boy recliner, surrounded by plastic flowers and candlesticks in his mother Leta's wood-paneled house. Leta is ninety-three years old, and Richard has been living with her for the past twelve years, ever since he retired from the ministry. Here he sleeps for eighteen hours a day, sometimes plays a little piano, and watches TV. He tells me that when he has a doctor's appointment, a therapy session, or a visit from a friend, he can spend the entire day just getting ready. He'll wake up midmorning, weary still, and take a couple of hours to muster the energy to shower. By the time he's dressed, it's already past lunchtime. "I used to be so active," he adds with a sigh. Now a visit such as mine will wipe him out completely.

In 2008, Richard noticed that his tennis game wasn't as good as he'd have liked—his knees were letting him down—and he decided to seek an elective knee replacement, a routine procedure performed thousands of times a day all over the world. He should have been discharged and walking on crutches within the week, back on the tennis court in three months, but he developed a serious lung infection after the surgery. He landed in the ICU, on a ventilator and intubated for four weeks. When he finally made it out of the hospital, his life had completely changed. He had to move in with his mother, something he thought would be temporary, but he never made it back to his own home. He couldn't function alone—he couldn't remember simple directions, when to take his medications, where he'd parked his car.

"The most difficult thing was the brain jumble," Richard says. It still is. When he tells a story, it can be as if his mind prevents him from remembering the most important parts. "The whole thing ends up sounding nonsensical." That doesn't work for delivering sermons to his congregation or counseling the needy one-on-one. He had no choice but to retire from the job he loved. He was only fifty-three, younger than I am now, and his once-full life became smaller, piece by piece.

"I felt like I'd been abandoned by God," he says. "My life, I just . . . I couldn't think. Process anything. It's still . . ." He pauses, looking for the words, his mouth opening once or twice as if he's found them. "Still kinda difficult. It really ticks me off." He shakes his head. He's in tears now, his frustration palpable in the humid room.

Richard's daughter, Ashleigh, once told me, "He has the memory he used to have, but the ability to execute is lost. It's as if a former master chess player is sitting in front of a chessboard. He knows that he knows how to play chess, but looking at this board with all of the pieces, he can't recall the rules, or even the name of the game."

Richard is living with post-intensive care syndrome (PICS), a debilitating condition composed of "neck-up" brain problems and "neck-down" body problems that survivors of critical illness often experience after a stay in the ICU. Though I didn't know it at the time, Teresa Martin was the first patient with PICS I ever saw. I imagine her life turned out something like Richard's, but I don't know for sure. I haven't been able to track her down. Today, millions of people around the world are struggling with PICS, some of them survivors of COVID-19. Most don't have any idea that they have a very real condition, and almost all have little access to the medical resources they need to cope with it. Few nurses and doctors outside the ICU world have even heard of PICS, much less the public at large.

The most striking point about PICS is that patients are not experiencing the residual effects of the original health problems that necessitated their admission to an ICU in the first place; instead, these are new conditions brought on by the lifesaving treatment they received. The brain problems—such as those Richard has—can be thought of as an ICU-acquired dementia, and the physical disability as an ICU-acquired muscle-and-nerve disease. PICS can also show up as mental health issues, primarily depression and post-traumatic stress disorder (PTSD). Those suffering with the condition include the young and the old. They come from low, middle, and high socioeconomic circumstances and from across a wide range of educational backgrounds.

In the United States and Europe alone, tens of millions of people are admitted annually to ICUs, with one half to three-quarters of survivors suffering from newly acquired cognitive, psychiatric, and/or physical impairments for many years after discharge. While the most severe forms of PICS arise in people admitted to ICUs for emergencies, it also occurs in patients, such as Richard, who develop complications after elective procedures. Most patients and their families—and many doctors, too—consider discharge from an ICU as the victorious end to a struggle against critical illness, but often the hardest part of a patient's experience is just beginning.

Time and again during the COVID-19 pandemic, I saw videos of balloon-laden celebrations as coronavirus survivors were discharged, often after weeks or months in the hospital. Survival is something to be celebrated, but I worried, thinking about what might be in store, even an hour later, when they arrived home and couldn't get up a step or two or remember basics about their former life. Like other survivors, they seemed oblivious that they were about to experience a new normal. That their lives might be changed forever. Survival may have come at a big cost, and sometimes people may not even feel "lucky to be alive," despite everyone telling them it's so.

• • •

I wonder how Richard felt when he realized his life would never again be what it once was. I first met him at a post-ICU support session organized through our Critical Illness, Brain Dysfunction, and Survivorship (CIBS) Center at Vanderbilt, which I founded twenty years ago and now codirect with my colleague Dr. Pratik Pandharipande. We have over ninety medical professionals, focused on research and ongoing care for people affected by critical illness. The weekly get-togethers and counseling sessions for survivors are spearheaded by neuropsychologist Dr. James "Jim" Jackson and intensivist (ICU doctor) Dr. Carla Sevin.

Most of the people in the group—including Richard—were not my patients in the ICU but made their way to us afterward for support. Some are local to Nashville, while others call in from across the country, or even from overseas on Zoom. Seeing patients beyond the bubble of the ICU is a healthy move for critical care. They still need us after discharge, and they need each other's support, too. When I first saw Richard, he was sitting at the long conference table, laughing, talking to Sarah Beth Miller, another ICU survivor, whom I'd known for years. I'd later learn that it takes Richard two to three times the normal amount of time to get to the support sessions as he drives the long way around the city, avoiding the stress of navigating the busy interstate and downtown. The time and day of the meetings have carefully been chosen so attendees can avoid rush hour traffic. The need to drive with extra caution is part of everyone's new normal.

From across the table, I'd caught fragments of Richard and Sarah Beth's conversation as it bounced from the Oscars to the Pulitzers, from their childhoods and onto the vagaries of current life. Nowhere could I sense any cognitive difficulties. No one would ever have known that they were suffering, or that they felt embarrassed and impaired, worried that their brain might betray them at any moment. Only later, as Richard spoke to the group, trying to answer a specific question, did I notice the brain jumble. He had told me it could come on suddenly. His sentences were convoluted and freewheeling, circling around the point. It was as if he were avoiding the interstate again, taking every side road in sight and endlessly trying to loop back. It was excruciating to listen to him. I began to understand his pain.

He wears a well-pressed shirt and a tie to the support group, his going-out attire, but here in his house he's dressed in a faded navy hoodie. He looks haggard. I figure it's time to call it a day and get up to leave. Glancing into the cluttered kitchen, I see a case of A&W diet root beer, which Richard says gets him through the day.

"Oh, wait." He moves toward his piano. "Do you want me to play for you?" He pulls out the bench and sits down, a large smile spreading across his face. He tilts his head toward me as I stand in the doorway, light from the setting sun brightening the wooden paneling and his framed awards from bygone days. The piano clanks a little, out of tune, but Richard's voice rings out, sending the words skyward: "I see the stars, I hear the rolling thunder. . . ." I wonder if he's remembering his days as a missionary or if he's just happy to hold on to the here and now. I pause, listening to his heart-lifting song, struck all over again by the raw courage of survivors. Their ability to reconfigure the pieces of their shattered lives.

• • •

I've known Sarah Beth Miller since 2003, when her ICU doctor referred her to Dr. Jackson and me for neuropsychological testing. With short gray hair and a dimpled smile, Sarah Beth radiates positivity. She grew up around horses on a farm in Goodlettsville, not so far from Nashville, and is well versed in getting right back on the horse that throws you. She's in my office, telling me about the recent passing of her mother. She speaks with eloquence and verve, her eyes bright with tears but also joy. She's not one to dwell on sadness.

Sarah Beth's story is both unique and familiar, one of critical illness emerging out of the blue and pushing a life off track. When she landed in the ICU on May 27, 2002, everything was humming along nicely. She was thirty years into a career with the phone company, one of the first female engineers hired by South Central Bell in Tennessee, and still there when it became AT&T. She was looking forward to a relaxing Memorial Day weekend. Instead, after struggling with a high fever and exhaustion, she was brought to the emergency department, where she collapsed, unconscious.

Over the next twelve hours, Sarah Beth developed pneumonia, sepsis, and acute respiratory distress syndrome (ARDS). Her lungs filled with fluid, and her heart and kidneys started to fail. She was raced to the ICU and placed on life support, attached to a ventilator and sedated. She almost died. She fluctuated between coma and delirium, hallucinating, scared, and confused. Her next clear memories were of fireworks celebrations, heard from her room on July 4. She'd been in the ICU for over five weeks.

When Sarah Beth was put in touch with Dr. Jackson and me, about a year after her discharge, she said something was very wrong with her. She just didn't know what. She'd spent the first few months after her near-death experience recovering at home, trying to regain her strength. "I couldn't even pick up a fork," she said. Her mother moved in with her. There was no other way she could survive. They corralled her sister Diane and brother Ken to help with the day-to-day. Sarah Beth received physical therapy, but it didn't help much, and getting up and down even a few stairs proved Herculean.

After three months, Sarah Beth figured she should head back to work. It's what was expected of her; she'd been in the hospital and now she was out; she'd been sick, she'd survived, and it was time to move on. She mustered the courage and physical energy to head back to her job, ready to pick up where she'd left off. But it wasn't that simple.

"The first day at the office," Sarah Beth explained, "I turned the computer on, looked at some stuff, and thought, 'Hmm, I wonder what I'm supposed to do.' I called my workmate Donna. 'Well,' she said, 'just run your reports.' 'What reports?' I asked." Sarah Beth had studied differential equations, complex numbers, and math theory in college. At the telephone company she'd been recognized as an expert in complicated engineering concepts. Now she could barely remember what her job was.

Sarah Beth started to work from home, eventually getting through her workday—one that used to take her eight hours—by starting at six in the morning and finishing at about ten at night.

Her main obstacle was difficulty focusing. She just didn't have an attention span anymore. A fly in the room might distract her, or a noise outside, and she'd spend fifteen minutes thinking about that instead of working. Before her ICU stay, she'd been an avid reader, taking a book along everywhere she went. "But after, I'd be reading and might see the word *black* and think, 'Well, that doesn't make sense.' So I'd read it again and the word is *back*, not *black*. I couldn't get through anything because that happened with every sentence. The words just didn't make sense."

When Dr. Jackson and I met her at the CIBS Center, Sarah Beth needed answers. She told us about her weakness and exhaustion, and the way she had to work sixteen-hour days just to get by. That she felt like a different person. And the worst of it, that no one seemed to think she was still sick. That much I understood. She seemed perfectly well to me, too.

First, Sarah Beth underwent a two-hour neuropsychological battery with Dr. Jackson testing her with components of the Wechsler Adult Intelligence Scale. When we all sat down afterward to go through the results, her first question was "What's my IQ?" She seemed so eager to know. That wasn't something we usually focused on as it's not the best gauge of how a person will perform in daily life tasks such as driving, working, and getting through the day.

"Oh, it's good," said Dr. Jackson, glancing at the papers. "It's above average. In the 110 range."

"What?" exclaimed Sarah Beth. She looked upset. "I was always around 140!"

I stared at her. That was a massive difference. It turned out she'd had her IQ tested many times before as part of her job.

"Well, no wonder I can't get through my work anymore," she added quietly.

Her drop in IQ was catastrophic. As Dr. Jackson explained, IQ on cognitive tests should be quite stable over time since the results are age adjusted. Even if she had lost a step in her brain function as part of normal senescence compared to when she was in her twenties and thirties, her IQ should have stayed roughly the same. I knew that every 15 points on an IQ test equals one standard deviation from normal—adjusted for age, education, and sex—and so Sarah Beth's drop of nearly 30 points would be commensurate with a person of average IQ (a score of 100) dropping down two standard deviations to a score of 70, which represents intellectual disability. Sarah Beth was highly cognitively impaired for her, and she knew it. She took off her glasses and slowly rubbed the lenses with the edge of her blouse.

Later, Sarah Beth told me that this was the instant she realized how much she'd lost. She'd known something was wrong—she was a math major who couldn't balance her checkbook anymore—but she hadn't realized the full extent of her cognitive decline. Now she had a number that documented this, and that resonated with her. She remembered who she used to be and saw the distance between her former self and this new version. It was a desolate realization.

I've since seen this moment many times, when people regard the chasm between their life before and after an ICU stay. When they question if it was worth it. I tried to imagine what it was like for math whiz Sarah Beth, who had coasted through complicated equations, to develop life-threatening pneumonia and then celebrate a survival that left her unable to remember even the most basic aspects of a job she'd excelled at for decades. Especially when everyone she knew was shrugging and saying she seemed fine. For Sarah Beth, this was the hardest part of her post-ICU survival: living with an illness that was invisible to her friends, family, colleagues, and even her doctors.

• • •

It's been over fifteen years since Sarah Beth came home from the ICU. Unable to manage the grueling sixteen-hour workdays, she ended up retiring at age fifty-two, more than a decade earlier than she'd planned, and has created a different life for herself—smaller in some aspects, but Sarah Beth refuses to see it that way. She came up with a fairly aggressive regimen of sudoku, Scrabble, and word jumbles, and, yes, she started reading again. She believes this "brain rehab," as she calls it, has helped her rewire her neural pathways. When I ask her what advice she has for those struggling after an ICU stay, she is quick to answer, "Don't live in the past or the future. And find something you're passionate about." For her, volunteering at a horseback-riding program for special-needs children has kept her busy. "Did you know that Winston Churchill said, 'There is something about the outside of a horse that is good for the inside of a man'?" she asks. I didn't. She then tells me about a three-year-old girl with severe autism who rarely spoke yet during her first riding session called out, "Ma!"

"We couldn't believe it! We all started crying." Sarah Beth pauses. "Nothing like that ever happened at the phone company."

I've noticed that it's the patients, such as Sarah Beth, who accept where and who they are today (even if they don't like it) who make the most progress in recovery. Additionally, those who feel they have found others "like them," who can identify with their suffering, are able not only to increase tolerance of their situation but also cultivate authentic acceptance over time. My daughter Blair introduced me to Viktor Frankl's *Man's Search for Meaning*, his book about his experiences as a prisoner in Nazi concentration camps. It has helped me understand the value of survivors' ability to reframe their situation, to narrow the stifling gap between their expected and actual quality of life. To find new meaning for themselves.

• • •

In October 2012 in Sacramento, I gave a talk to hundreds of hospital administrators, physicians, and nurses on ways to enhance patient care in the ICU and thereby improve their post-ICU lives (see "Resources for Patients, Families, Caregivers, and Medical Professionals"). While there, I heard Anthony Russo, a critical care survivor, speak about his experience of life after the ICU. He detailed his daily struggles with cognitive impairment, depression, and anxiety. It was textbook PICS. Life turned upside down by an unexpected ICU admission. In Anthony's case, he'd been in the prime of life, running five miles a day, when he sat next to a man with the sniffles at a board meeting. It was 2009 and Anthony caught H1N1 influenza. In less than a day, the virus had attacked his entire body the way a burst pipe can quickly flood a house, making the interior of his lungs leaky and fill with water, dropping his blood pressure into shock, causing him not to get enough blood to his kidneys and brain, leaving him on a ventilator, on dialysis, and in delirium for weeks. Afterward, his life was forever changed.

A couple of years after the Sacramento conference, Anthony and his wife, Debra, came to Nashville to see me at the CIBS Center. He was really struggling, and they were worried their marriage was falling apart. Anthony alternated between silence and anger, and Debra felt pushed away. She didn't know how to help him. As we talked, they both echoed something that stunned me. The first time they had ever heard of PICS was when I spoke about it at the conference. Though Anthony had stood up and told a packed room full of strangers about the way his life had become unmanageable after his stay in an ICU, he hadn't known he was suffering from an illness. One that accounted for all his symptoms. He must have told his story to many health professionals, and no one had enlightened him. Had we failed so badly as critical care doctors to teach people about PICS, beyond our bubble of ICU meetings and specialized journals?

In 2019, I spoke in Sacramento again, at a Hospital Quality Institute conference. There, onstage beside me, stood Anthony and Debra

Russo to inform and educate the audience on the devastation that comes from living with PICS. My daughter Brooke attended the conference with me, and afterward the Russos invited us for dinner. Their home is a picture-perfect house on a seventy-acre vineyard just south of Napa. They own construction and real estate businesses, and their grape production is booming. Every season their vineyard yields about eight tons of grapes per acre, the reds going to Francis Ford Coppola's cabernet sauvignon, and the whites to Emmolo.

We sat down for dinner in a courtyard surrounded by carved stonework and perfectly manicured walls of ivy—Anthony, Debra, their grown-up daughter, Riley, her husband, Jeff, their young son, Max, and Brooke and me. It was a beautiful evening, and we were served a bountiful meal of fresh greens, lemon chicken, risotto, and fruit cobbler, with a bottle of cabernet made from their own grapes. The Russos seemed to be living their dream, achieved through years of hard work. But I knew that just below the surface their life was extraordinarily difficult.

Ten years after his ICU experience, Anthony still suffers from excruciating depression. He's told me he has days when he wishes he'd never survived. That it wasn't worth it, and all he wants to do is give up. Like many other ICU survivors, he suffers from PTSD, perceived as feelings of mortal threat, as if he's surrounded by a pervasive danger he can't fully grasp. For many survivors, their PTSD is tied to the delirium dreams they had while on life support. Many of these dreams are violent, and in some the brain tries to make sense of routine medical procedures—having an MRI, the insertion of a catheter—and turns them into scenarios of harm. Delirium dreams feel like lived experiences and are extremely difficult to shake. Anthony is terrified to sleep, as he knows the dreams will come back to him, except he doesn't refer to them as dreams. "They were events," he told me. Events in which he fails to save his daughter, Riley, and watches her die right in front of him, again and again. Events that still run through his brain most nights.

About one in five ICU survivors develops PTSD, and one in three develops depression and anxiety. This psychological damage often exacerbates physical and cognitive impairments, making it even harder for survivors to leave their homes to socialize, run errands, or return to work. Subsequent feelings of isolation and failure compound the problem. More than half of patients suffering with PICS haven't returned to work a year after their ICU discharge.

During dinner, amid the chatter and laughter, Anthony sometimes rose from his seat and paced or disappeared into the kitchen. It was as if he could never truly relax. I wondered if he had a form of akathisia, as if a motor were running inside him that wouldn't turn off, but it was probably anxiety. He was wound so tight. Every time he left his seat, I noticed Debra's eyes follow him, checking on him. His struggles clearly impacted his whole family. We see this over and over, the loved ones of survivors pulled into an ever-widening vortex of loss and pain, sometimes developing depression, anxiety, and PTSD themselves. It's a family disease, and we refer to it as PICS-F (for "family"). Many families don't survive the effects of PICS intact. Marriages end in divorce, siblings quarrel, and friends turn away, unable to cope. I'm glad that, despite their troubles, the Russos still have one another.

As the sun went down and our dinner drew to a close, little Max clambered onto his grandfather's lap, the only one oblivious to his pain. I watched as they snuggled together, and I hoped that for this moment, Anthony's torment was cast aside. That he felt good to be alive.

• • •

As a critical care doctor, it's hard for me to acknowledge that Richard Langford, Sarah Beth Miller, and Anthony Russo all suffer from a set of brain and body diseases that emerged while they were in the ICU and still persist today, over ten years later. As doctors, we thought we were doing our jobs, saving lives that would decades earlier surely have been lost. Our only goal was to help our patients, yet now we see the harm that happened, too. While the work we do at the CIBS Center can alleviate their suffering, it doesn't come close to eliminating it. There are always going to be, for them and their loved ones, residual pains and ongoing challenges.

Richard, Sarah Beth, and Anthony are products of an old-school critical care culture that focused on saving lives at all costs, one that normalized keeping ventilated patients deeply sedated, paralyzed with medications, and often delirious, immobilized in their hospital beds, and isolated from family and friends. In retrospect, we couldn't have created a better environment for causing PICS if we'd tried. As a young doctor, I'd wanted to make a difference and save lives. It turns out I should have taken my thinking one step further and considered what kind of life a survivor would be facing. That was a journey that would take me over twenty years.

Chapter 2

Early History of Critical Care—Bumpy Gravel Roads to ICU Interstates

I was taught that the way of progress was neither swift nor easy.

—Marie Curie, *Pierre Curie*

ONE SUMMER WEEKEND I hiked with my family to Clingmans Dome in Tennessee's Smoky Mountains, following the river's chatter through the woods, then stepping out into highland meadows. This immersion in nature helps clear my mind. The lurking threat (usually unfulfilled) of seeing a bear provides some excitement, and the summit always takes me by surprise. This time was no exception, and my chest lifted slightly as I gazed at distant mountains almost a hundred miles away. Despite the day's sweltering heat, it was chilly at the top, and I was reminded of how the weather can change in minutes. I felt like a speck in this vast universe of ours, but also incredibly alive, so rooted in the here and now.

As we headed down, a rainstorm came out of nowhere and soaked us through. We hurried down the path toward shelter in the woods. When we were finally out of the downpour, we stopped and took stock of our dripping hair and faces, our clothes plastered to our skin, our soggy, squeaking boots. We laughed, made giddy by adrenaline, by the sheer force of nature, by our helplessness within its grasp.

The thrill I get in the ICU is different. I still feel it after all these years as the heavy doors swing open and I walk in. At the hospital, I am ready to stave off whatever nature throws at me. When critical illness strikes out of the blue, I will not easily submit. As I start my day, I'm aware that my life is about to intersect with many others. Even now a patient may be on the way to my care, wheeled in on a gurney, having the worst day of her life. My role is to find the best way to help her. A sense of urgency, the excitement and threat of bear, follows everything we do, even when there is no overt code blue. A feeling that something is always about to happen, and we need to be ready. Being an intensivist means thinking, "How can our team defeat death today and turn our patient toward life?"

As I enter the COVID unit, I'm especially aware of the fierce battle we're waging against an evolving virus sending its death toll higher and higher, while we push back. We have a slew of patients on dialysis and ventilators, and several on extracorporeal membrane oxygenation (ECMO) machines as well. Even with the help of ventilators, their lungs are struggling, too damaged with pneumonia to exchange oxygen and carbon dioxide. ECMO does it for them, taking the blood out of their bodies and "refueling" it before returning it through the veins. Machines are lined up inside and outside the patients' rooms, two or three deep in places, our armament against this deadly disease, with legions of nurse practitioners, nurses, pharmacists, respiratory therapists, physical and occupational therapists, and doctors everywhere, barely recognizable in their protective gear. We are mobilized. It's impossible for me not to think in military metaphors.

It's late morning and I see the nurse practitioner team looking wholly exasperated and moving quickly, responding to yet another unforeseen clinical downturn. Their patient just popped a lung and needs an emergency surgical chest tube.

A doctor is shaking her head. "Look at his chest X-ray with that huge pneumo."

I nod. A glance at the image shows that one lung has collapsed, and when I turn to see the patient, I'm not surprised that he's struggling to breathe. The COVID patients suffer so many unexpected complications. It's as if their bodies are under attack from all sides. We leap in with our interventions and fix one problem, only to have something else occur the second we turn our backs.

In recent weeks, our patients' lungs have failed, then their kidneys, and their brains. As if that weren't enough, several developed an unusual pattern of air leaking inside their besieged bodies. It's something I've rarely seen to such an extent. Our three current patients with this subcutaneous emphysema are deformed by air seeping throughout their chest, abdomen, and even their face, their eyelids and genitalia puffed up with air, beyond recognition. For a moment, I think it's almost a blessing that their loved ones can't visit and witness the destruction that COVID has wrought, but then I dismiss the thought. Families are desperate to see loved ones, especially when they are so gravely ill.

As a young physician, I thought the body's organ compartments were discrete, but in fact the human body is like one of those old mansions in the movies, riddled with secret trapdoors and passages that allow escape without notice. I learned this one night years ago, as I was closing in on my ten thousand hours of emergency-medicine coverage and thought this time spent honing a skill assured me of expert status. A young man came in complaining of chest pain, so I ordered an EKG and X-ray and moved on to the next patient. When the data came back, I pulled up the imaging and saw air around his heart. I was confused. "Sir, what did you say you did today?" I asked. "Nothing other than go to the dentist!" The dentist had used an air-turbine drill to remove a tooth, and it dawned on me the air must have jetted into the man's gums, down through secret passageways of his neck, and all the way into his chest and around his heart. I assured him he'd be fine as the air

29

would reabsorb on its own and checked on him the next day to be sure I was right.

Unfortunately for our three COVID patients, their outcome is not so simple. The amount of air escaping through trapdoors is at a dangerous level, misshaping their bodies with every whoosh from their ventilators. It also indicates that they are very, very sick. When the condition first showed up in our COVID-ICU, we considered how best to resolve it, whether it was even possible to do so. We consulted with thoracic surgeon Dr. Matthew Bacchetta, and in one of those "Oh, by the way" conversations that happen so often in medicine, it turned out that he'd seen this rare issue before, back in New York years ago. He'd used a technique called gill slits to deal with it. Learning from him, that's what we do now. Two incisions in the patient's skin, above the nipples, to allow just enough of the leaking air to escape slowly back into the atmosphere. Another invasive procedure. Another battle won. Or maybe just a skirmish. For now.

• • •

If you walk into an intensive care unit in many accredited acute care hospitals today, you will witness something that's easy to take for granted. What used to be, as recently as fifteen years ago, a row of small, dingy rooms with cumbersome machinery has become a spacious set of bright and shiny suites, geared up with a multitude of technologically advanced tools worth well over a million dollars. A world away from the open ICU with its chipped metal beds at Charity Hospital. When war breaks out inside the human body, this equipment is exquisitely tuned to fight, one patient at a time. It costs about $2,000 to $4,000 per square foot to build a modern ICU room in the United States. A room at the Ritz would be closer to $400 per square foot, making a fully loaded ICU room perhaps the most "luxurious" bedroom on the planet, even before factoring in the cost of salaries of the health-care team, medicine, meals, and other aspects of daily care such as labs, fluids, radiology, and life support. A stay there might last a week and costs on average $100,000.

A critically ill patient with failing organs cared for in such a room might end up on the receiving end of everything that modern medicine has to offer: advanced around-the-clock computerized monitoring, multiple central IV lines, feeding tubes, catheters, a breathing tube and mechanical ventilator, kidney dialysis, ultrasound, MRI imaging, and a vast array of medications, delivered from a rack of pumps that looks like a flight panel on a jet plane. Without the interventions of these machines and technology, the patient's vital organs would likely shut down and his life would end. But more and more often these days in critical care, we manage to keep death at bay.

In the United States alone, we spend more than $3 trillion on health care annually, and over the next decade that figure is projected to rise to approximately one-fifth of our entire GDP. That's compared to an average expenditure of just one-tenth of the GDP in other industrialized countries. Over the past two decades, we have doubled the amount spent on critical care to over $100 billion, and that figure is sure to increase. Interestingly, while the overall number of hospital beds across the nation has stayed flat, the proportion of these that are ICU beds has steadily escalated. As medical expertise and lifesaving technologies develop, more and more critically ill patients end up in the hospital, whereas their medical conditions would once have led to certain death at home or in nursing homes. Now, with our extraordinary fixes and even cures, patients turn up in the ICU in droves, ready for a continued shot at life.

Some extremely sick patients receive increasingly complex care in hospital wards outside the ICU as lifesaving technology has grown smaller in size, more commonplace, and more easily used by a larger array of health-care professionals. Within ICUs, patients on the brink of death are cared for in well over one hundred thousand intensive care beds each day, in around three thousand hospitals across the country. These patients now spend over 25 million days in ICUs in the United States, and the global figure is even more staggering.

As the number of critically ill patients has expanded around the world, we, as a medical community, have become better at saving lives. From 1988 to 2012, we accomplished a one-third reduction in the likelihood of death for ICU patients. Sepsis is the leading reason people are admitted emergently to an ICU. With this condition, the immune system overreacts to a bacterial, viral, or fungal infection and causes multiple organs to fail. In 2000, over 60 percent of patients died if they developed refractory septic shock, which is when the cardiovascular system collapses so profoundly that blood pressure must be buoyed with liters of intravenous fluid and medications to avoid immediate death. Through decades of work in sepsis by hundreds of global scientists and investigative teams—led by colleagues such as Dr. Derek Angus in Pittsburgh, Dr. Kathy Rowan in London, Dr. Jean-Louis Vincent in Brussels, Dr. John Marshall in Toronto, and Dr. Simon Finfer in Sydney—by 2020 that number was cut in half with about 30 percent of patients dying from septic shock. Over this same period of progress, in the midst of our constant drive toward more and more complex lifesaving interventions, we began asking ourselves some crucial questions. Should saving lives be a doctor's prime focus in the ICU? Is this really our best marker of success?

• • •

It can be hard to fathom that the field of critical care—so ordinary to us now as we watch it play out on our favorite TV shows—is a fairly recent newcomer to the long and rich history of medicine and has its beginnings just over 150 years ago. During the Crimean War, in the 1850s, British nurse and health-care reformer Florence Nightingale requested that the most seriously ill patients be placed closer to the nurses' station so they could be monitored more attentively. This is the essence of critical care: the sickest patients being treated in a separate and specific place. By the mid-1920s, neurosurgeon Walter Dandy had started a specialized twenty-four-hour nursing unit for critically ill postoperative surgical patients at Johns Hopkins Hospital, a forerunner of modern intensive care units. During World War II, in Italy and North Africa, dedicated shock units were used to resuscitate large numbers of severely injured soldiers. In 1942, in Boston, after the infamous Cocoanut Grove nightclub fire, Massachusetts General Hospital created a makeshift burn unit within hours to care for thirty-nine critically ill survivors. Around the same time, the Mayo brothers in Rochester, Alton Ochsner in New Orleans at Charity (which I came to know so well decades later), and physicians at New York Hospital all established large recovery rooms for those undergoing increasingly complex surgeries such as the removal of lungs, stomach, and the esophagus. Setting up rooms specifically for the sickest patients proved extremely wise and yielded a doubling in patient survival. But not until the 1970s did such rooms become commonplace in US hospitals.

At first, specialized recovery rooms were a place to oversee and monitor gravely ill patients more easily. As medical technology grew exponentially, they became a place both for the sickest patients and for the lifesaving machines that would treat them. In many ways, the evolution of critical care runs parallel to the advances in modern technology—and not always in the best interest of the patients.

While I was in college, I read *Diffusion of Innovations* by Everett Rogers and became fascinated by his theory of the way innovations take hold and are adopted over time until they become mainstream. Rogers devised different categories: innovators, early adopters, early majority, late majority, and laggards, and I started to view the world around me through this lens. I realized that Marvin Lessman, owner of the produce farm where I'd worked as a planter and picker, was a classic early adopter, driving south every spring to the Rio Grande

Valley in Texas to buy up early-growing okra and tomato plants and newer types of seed with higher yields, to get a jump on his competition. I'd gone with him on several occasions and listened to him explain his strategy. It worked. Our vegetable crops were usually the biggest for miles around. Once I'd learned this theory, I saw it in play frequently and never more so than in medicine. Innovators and early adopters have constantly urged us forward, reaching new frontiers at an astonishing rate.

The advent of the ventilator is just one such example. As the COVID-19 pandemic highlighted, this lifesaving machine is a mainstay of any modern-day ICU, saving millions of patients from certain death each year. Yet a machine with the ability to breathe for a patient whose lungs are too damaged to do so—and to buy time for the patient's body to recover—is a fairly recent invention. At the end of the nineteenth century, rudimentary ventilators helped patients breathe, but these machines were a far cry from today's ventilators. They often enclosed patients in a box and used bellows to expand the chest and pull air into the lungs. These so-called negative-pressure ventilators evolved over the next forty years and reached their pinnacle with the iron lung, invented by Philip Drinker and Louis Agassiz Shaw Jr. in 1928, and used during the polio epidemics of the 1940s and '50s. Astounding photographs from the time show gymnasium-size wards filled with row upon row of these contraptions, enabling dozens of polio patients to breathe. With their help, death rates among polio patients with respiratory failure dropped dramatically, an extraordinary achievement.

Successful as they were, these iron lungs were not the precursors of the positive-pressure breathing machines in use today. Those were developed before the 1950s but not widely used until a polio epidemic in Denmark, where the number of infected and suffocating patients rapidly exceeded the number of available iron lungs. As the adage goes, necessity is the mother of invention, and when a new disease emerges or an old disease takes on a new twist, medicine must quickly adapt. In

Copenhagen, with dozens of people dying and just one iron lung in the entire city, anesthesiologist Dr. Bjørn Ibsen, another innovator and early adopter, came up with a radical solution.

In the summer of 1952, Copenhagen's polio epidemic ballooned to nine hundred patients. Of the first few dozen patients admitted with respiratory paralysis to the Blegdams Hospital, twenty-seven were dead within seventy-two hours, many of them drowning in their own phlegm as the polio virus attacked their nerves and stopped them from breathing. Blegdams's medical director, Dr. Henry Lassen, found himself under siege as his medical staff struggled desperately, at war without weapons. His colleague Dr. Mogens Bjørneboe had an idea. He urged Lassen, his boss, to consult Dr. Bjørn Ibsen, who was temporarily working at Blegdams. But Lassen's mind-set, shared by most physicians in the strict hierarchy of Danish medicine, was stuck in prewar days. He'd been at the helm for thirteen years and wasn't about to yield to an upstart with odd ideas. Instead, he called in his own friends as consultants, and the epidemic continued to rage.

However, Bjørneboe was convinced that Ibsen could provide a solution. Two years earlier, on a ship from New York to Denmark, Bjørneboe had met Doris Ibsen, who was returning from Boston. She'd explained to Bjørneboe how excited her husband, Bjørn Ibsen, was to be working in the anesthesia department at Massachusetts General, joining this fledgling field that had only recently been accredited in Denmark. On completing his training, Ibsen had returned to Denmark. In June 1952, Bjørneboe needed assistance on a difficult case with an infant paralyzed by tetanus, and with Lassen away on a short holiday, he had reached out to the anesthesiologist. Ibsen used curare, a toxic extract derived from plants, to relax the baby's muscles and placed a tube in his windpipe to manually breathe for him. The infant died, but when the polio epidemic raged later in the summer, Bjørneboe again thought of Ibsen. Tetanus. Polio. The similarities were there.

Eventually Bjørneboe convinced Lassen to allow Ibsen to study the records and autopsies of the polio patients, and to come up with a potential solution. And he did: cut a hole in the patients' trachea (windpipe) and insert a tube to allow doctors to blow air directly *into* the body with positive pressure, rather than pull the chest wall outward with negative pressure applied inside an iron lung. When presented with the idea, Lassen doubted it would work, but in an act of immense humility, he acquiesced, and Ibsen's theory was tested.

In August, a twelve-year-old girl, Vivi Ebert, was admitted to Blegdams Hospital with respiratory paralysis. The virus had invaded her brain stem and spinal cord in a way that left her suffocating. According to Ibsen and Lassen, she was "in a very bad condition, with paralysis of all four extremities. She . . . was gasping for breath and drowning in her own secretions, cyanotic and sweating." Death for her was certain. She became the index patient into whose trachea they inserted the breathing tube. Attached to the tube was a rubber bag filled with an oxygen supply, and by squeezing it, Ibsen blew air into her body. This is known as bag ventilation. Initially, she struggled, went into a coma, and nearly died, and other physicians left the scene thinking the end was near. Out of desperation, Ibsen gave her 100 mg of the anesthetic Pentothal. Immediately, her fighting stopped, and by squeezing the bag of air, the doctors were able to breathe for her. They saved her life. Vivi Ebert became one of the first people ever to survive through positive-pressure ventilation. A new approach to respiratory failure took hold, and critical care medicine leaped forward.

With the tracheostomy approach deemed a success, Ibsen and Lassen could treat the other polio patients at Blegdams. They did so, taking care of them all in a newly created specialized section of the hospital. The only problem left was how to ensure that air would continue to fill the lungs once the tube was inserted into the windpipe. In an extraordinary show of community care, over the next few months, approximately fifteen hundred medical and dental students from the University of Copenhagen sat at the bedsides of the tracheotomized patients and manually bag-ventilated them throughout the day and night, forcing air into their lungs until they were strong enough to breathe on their own. Despite the magnitude of the public health disaster, by mid-November the mortality rate for polio patients with respiratory failure had plummeted from 87 percent to 31 percent.

Ibsen's and Bjørneboe's forward thinking swept in huge changes in medicine and the role that machines and technology would play in patient care. Within a year in Stockholm, Sweden, when the next European polio epidemic struck, engineers and scientists built on Ibsen's lifesaving approach and raced to develop the first generation of positive-pressure ventilators. The machines ran on electricity and eliminated the need for manual bag-ventilation.

From these rudimentary beginnings in Copenhagen, we can draw a direct line to the fancy computerized ventilators found today in any top-notch ICU. In addition, Ibsen's separate hospital rooms, dedicated to his seriously ill respiratory patients, paved the way for hospitals in Denmark and beyond to set up spaces devoted entirely to critically ill patients.

I've always appreciated this story, the ingenuity and determination of the doctors in the face of an epidemic, the mobilization of the students to bag-ventilate the patients. But I especially like the serendipity of the meeting on the boat between Bjørneboe and Ibsen's wife, Doris, that eventually brought the two men together. As if it were just meant to be. This seems to happen often in medicine, in smaller and larger ways.

Only recently did I discover that while Vivi Ebert lived for twenty more years, read voraciously, painted watercolors, fell in love, and married, she left Blegdams as a quadriplegic and required the help of a ventilator for the rest of her life. Her fate doesn't make Ibsen's ingenuity any less impressive nor does it diminish the vital role that the 1952 Copenhagen polio epidemic played in advancing critical care medicine. Instead it reminds me that survivors of critical illness, those who struggle after their lives have been saved, are a central part of this narrative. Yet their stories are often invisible.

• • •

Innovations in critical care continued to boom. The years between 1940 and 1960 were an exciting time in medical technology as new inventions flooded into hospitals. The artificial kidney was created in 1944 and developed as a clinically usable machine in the 1960s. This was the era of the pacemaker, the heart-lung bypass machine, the ultrasound scanner, the defibrillator, and various renditions of the latest mechanical ventilator. These machines began to offer a variety of ways to dose oxygen and deliver breaths and came with alarms that alerted medical personnel to air-pressure problems. The wonder drug penicillin started to be mass-produced, and developments in knowledge about blood types and storage meant that blood could be collected and made available for transfusion in critically ill patients. Initially, these advances in blood banking were fueled by the large numbers of American soldiers serving in World War II. Dr. Charles Drew, a Black surgeon and medical researcher, created a means to process and preserve plasma (the liquid without the red blood cells), enabling it to be transported and stored until needed. He spearheaded a national blood-banking effort for the American Red Cross, encouraging Americans to donate blood to be processed into plasma as part of the war effort, leading to countless lives saved and to blood transfusions becoming customary in modern medical care.

As we note the tremendous march of progress, it's also important to acknowledge the shameful racial segregation and racism that occurred alongside: at first only white Americans were allowed to donate blood (meaning that Dr. Drew himself was forbidden), and then, after an outcry, Black donors were permitted, but only on a segregated basis. Blood was labeled "Caucasian" or "Negroid." This became standard practice and occurred throughout the US health-care system until the passage of the Civil Rights Act in 1964, and not until the late 1960s and early 1970s did Arkansas and Louisiana put an end to the practice.

As the century moved along, medical innovations abounded, and the first single-organ liver, lung, pancreas, and heart transplants took place. It was a good time to be a patient, as doctors swooped in to save lives with their newfangled technology. Doctors and nurses, swathed from head to toe in gowns, began to specialize in critical care medicine, drawn to this innovative field where they oversaw patients on the brink of death with the constant assistance of monitors and chirping alarms.

In the 1960s and '70s, people followed in Dr. Ibsen's footsteps by grouping patients and medical technology in specific sections of hospitals to provide intensive care around the clock, delivered by a new breed of physician, focused on critical care. Among the first of these modern units were those opened by Claude Bernard in Paris, Vladimir Alexandrovitch Negovsky in Moscow, Peter Safar and Ake Grenvik at Baltimore City Hospital and the University of Pittsburgh, and Max Harry Weil in Los Angeles at the University of Southern California. Doctors and the public alike embraced these specialized wards, and soon intensive care units were springing up in hospitals across the country.

By 1981, ICUs were in 95 percent of American hospitals. The face of health care had changed in an extraordinarily short time. Even the sickest patients could now survive potentially life-threatening conditions, when just ten or twenty years earlier they wouldn't have stood a chance. I'd witnessed this firsthand. One of my childhood best friends, a member of our summer book club and a fellow competitive swimmer, Stephen Teagle, was treated in the ICU on multiple occasions. Born with cystic fibrosis, an inherited disorder that damages the lungs, digestive system, and other organs, Stephen often developed severe infections that led to sepsis. He would end up in the ICU in downtown Shreveport, miss a few swim practices, and then be back, saved by critical care. We all took his absences and returns for granted, thought of his medical treatments as completely normal. We had no idea that if he'd been born just a decade earlier, he might not have made it to his fifth birthday.

The arrival of all this astonishing lifesaving machinery catalyzed a shift in thinking within the medical community. The Hippocratic oath doesn't explicitly call for physicians to save lives, yet they started to believe it was their job to do so, even in the most extreme circumstances. Now they had the tools to make it a reality, or at least the possibility lay within their grasp. This is the mind-set that drew me to the field in medical school. The doctors in the ICU were the ones who saved patients. They didn't let young mothers with newborn babies die, such as my patient Sarah Bollich. With their dazzling technology, they were a patient's final hope for evading death. I wanted to join their ranks.

• • •

In the fall of 1992, I was excited to write a letter to my mother telling her I was about to enter the fields of pulmonary (lung) and critical care. I'd completed my three years of residency in internal medicine at Wake Forest and was staying on there as a fellow to pursue three more years of training. I had fallen in love on the first day of medical school with Kim Adams, a young woman from New Jersey who had studied cancer cells at MIT, drawn to the beauty in the color patterns they made under her microscope. She was vibrant and fun, her eyes alight with curiosity about the world. We were married and living in Winston-Salem, two doctors starting out together. I felt like a grown-up. I had even found myself a mentor, Dr. Ed Haponik, director of clinical practice and research in the critical care division. I knew my mom would be pleased to read about this. She had been a mentor to so many of her high school students, inviting them over to our house on Mockingbird Lane, helping them learn lines from Shakespeare for the plays she directed. I was in grade school at the time and had loved to listen to their discussions. They seemed to know so much, and I hoped I would absorb their knowledge.

The next week my mom called me to say she had received my letter, asking for more details about my work, but I was running late for my clinic with Dr. Haponik. "I'm learning how to use life-support machines," I said. "To save people whose organs are failing from lots of different diseases. I'll have to call you back."

As Dr. Haponik's fellow, I saw the clinic patients first, usually people with chronic lung problems, and prepared a presentation for him so that together we could determine the best plan for their treatment. For new patients, especially, I tried to ready myself mentally for immersion into their lives, knowing that the medical history and the physical take a long time to complete. But that day, I felt rushed. I didn't have a chance to read the chart before entering the room, and as I opened the door to introduce myself to the first patient, I was startled. A woman greeted me, "Hello, Doctor, what a privilege it is to see you today." I couldn't speak. Nothing could have prepared me for this. It was Dr. Maya Angelou.

I'd never stopped thinking about *I Know Why the Caged Bird Sings* since my mother's summer book club fifteen years earlier, and now I was standing in front of the woman who, to me, defined grit and triumph over adversity. Her first memoir had inspired me to stand up for the underdog, to fight for the "pickers" with no voice. I took a breath, regained my composure, and began to ask about her, her medical story, and what had brought her to the hospital that day. I admitted that I had read her books, which drew a smile. Then I continued with the physical exam, listening to her heart, her lungs, checking her nail beds, observing her breathing cadence, and even the way she used the muscles of her neck on inhalation. Through my stethoscope I heard crackles at the base of her right lung, and when I inquired about her shortness of breath, she asked if she could demonstrate by singing. I almost fell over with gratitude. And sing she did, in a voice resonant and at times remarkably husky, though I noted her gasp for air at the end of each line.

41

During her visit that day, Dr. Angelou told Dr. Haponik and me that she was working on a special project—a poem that she would read at the inauguration of President Clinton—and she was concerned that her breathing problems might get worse. The only other poet in America's history to recite a poem at an inauguration had been Robert Frost, when he read for John F. Kennedy, over thirty years earlier. Frost had had trouble with his delivery that day because of the wind and a poor copy of the poem he'd written for the occasion, forcing him to go with an older poem, "The Gift Outright," which he knew by heart. Dr. Angelou wanted no such trouble, and Dr. Haponik and I were to be her physicians to ensure she had enough breath for success. We helped to tune up her breathing, recommended exercises to increase her lung capacity, and prescribed antibiotics to clear up a slight infection. We were in rarefied air that day.

I couldn't wait to call my mother at the end of the afternoon and tell her all about the visit. Dr. Angelou had given me permission to do so. As anchoring as ever, my mom came straight back to the advice she'd given me on my first day of medical school, saying, "Wes, I hope you remembered to look Dr. Angelou in the eye and talk directly to her as if she were the only person in the world who mattered to you at that moment." I was able to say that I had. That visit with Dr. Angelou was memorable to me for many reasons. Not least because it was one that epitomized for me how much I relished the patient-doctor interaction, the partnership we formed to find the best treatment path forward, one that worked for the patient's life. I didn't realize then how far I would be leaving this goal behind as I channeled myself into critical care. Nor how long it would take to get it back.

A few months later, in January 1993, I watched the presidential inauguration on television in great excitement. I felt a surge of pride as Dr. Angelou took the stage and delivered her moving poem "On the Pulse of Morning" with confidence, her words ringing out above the crowd. "Here on the pulse of this new day / You may have the grace to look up and out / . . . And say simply / Very simply / With hope / Good morning."

Her lungs seemed to be in fine shape. This once-voiceless woman could now be heard.

As the turn of the century approached, the world of medicine seemed to me to reflect her optimism. Having made great strides forward from simple beginnings, nothing could hold us back.

Chapter 3

Culture of Critical Care—The Era of Deep Sedation and Immobilization

> *Her mind tottered and slithered again, broke from its foundation and spun like a cast wheel in a ditch. . . . She sank easily through deeps and deeps of darkness until she lay like a stone at the farthest bottom of life. . . . The stench of corruption filled her nostrils. . . . She opened her eyes and saw pale light through a coarse white cloth over her face, knew that the smell of death was in her own body, and struggled to lift her hand.*

—Katherine Anne Porter, *Pale Horse, Pale Rider*, on her experience of delirium during the 1918 Spanish flu pandemic

A NURSE YELLED FOR assistance. Her patient was flatlining with oxygen levels down in the low 70s, and about ten of us rapidly filled the room. Near-death in the ICU always comes with a flurry of activity and noise, as alarms squawk and doctors issue commands. The team takes shape, machines are rushed in, and people position themselves around the patient to do their jobs.

As a young resident and fellow, at the first call of code blue I'd race to the head of the bed as the intubator, the person who puts the tube into the trachea to provide lifesaving air from the ventilator. But that day, my attending physician, Dr. Bob Chin, was already there so I stayed at the patient's feet and started assigning the different roles. Code leader was my second-favorite position when bedlam broke out. I reeled off everyone's names and positions: primary and backup on chest compressions, medication administration, recording times and drugs given, one to check for a pulse and another to draw blood for pH and gas levels, and, most important, one to bag the patient to get oxygen levels high again. It's all-hands-on-deck in a code, everyone moving toward the common purpose of not letting the patient die.

Dr. Chin called for the laryngoscope, a long metal blade that shines a light down into the throat and lifts the epiglottis, the cartilaginous flap just above the voice box. Once it's out of the way, we can see straight into the windpipe and slip the tube down past the tongue and vocal cords to a spot where the airway splits and goes to the lungs.

Even with bagging, our patient's oxygen levels were still only in the low 80s, and there was no time to waste. Dr. Chin pushed ahead with intubation. If you can get the tube into the trachea, everything changes for the better in a heartbeat. Like a car going off a cliff but, suddenly, a bridge appears and you can drive straight to the other side. I could feel the tension in the room, everyone on pins and needles, wanting the tube to start delivering air to the lungs, to see a rapid change in skin tone from blue to pink, and for the pulse oximeter readings to start rising. But it wasn't happening.

Dr. Chin lifted his arm toward the ceiling with the laryngoscope angled perfectly, then peered past the patient's lips. "I can't get the epiglottis out of the way," he said. "It's grade three and huge. I can't see the cords at all." A grade-three view happens only about one in a hundred times. It leaves you with no view of the glottis, which makes it much harder to get the tube into the trachea. "His oxygen's in the sixties, let's bag again," said the nurse. I made sure that all the meds were on board, that epi and atropine had both been given, and told the resident to resume CPR. But our patient's skin was turning blue again, his lips a deepening shade of purple. I could see the panic on Dr. Chin's face. That wasn't good—he was the one I always counted on to be calm during emergencies.

"I'm going to get this tube in!" He reached for the patient's jaws, thrust them skyward, repositioned the head, slipped the scope back into place, and lifted. "Damn epiglottis!" A senior nurse wiped huge beads of sweat off his forehead, away from his eyes. A person was dying in front of us. Dr. Chin was desperately focused and jabbed in the tube. "I got it!"

A medical student, applying pressure over the front of the patient's neck, exclaimed, "I felt it pass!" I moved a resident out of the way and, through my stethoscope, heard the air rush into both lungs. Everyone in the room began to breathe again, and we continued the code until the patient's heart was back in sinus rhythm and his blood pressure stabilized. It was harrowing and exhausting. I can still hear Dr. Chin's "I got it!" today, over twenty-five years later. Even now my heart quickens.

There's always a rush of emotion when you save someone's life. A collective exhale as the team registers just how close death had come, then a surge of excitement, and a swell of confidence. I noticed it especially as a young doctor. Not that I was under any illusions about being in control of life and death, but there was always a sense of satisfaction, of having perhaps played a small part in sending death scuttling.

During my seven years of training, between graduating medical school and becoming an attending physician, I kept a paper index card on each of my hospitalized patients for whom I was the primary doctor. I scribbled down details about them, their age, profession, diseases, labs, family members' names, even their dog's name, as well as any major medical events that occurred during my care. I don't know why I did it, other than maybe I felt the need for some tangible chronicle of my evolution as a physician—a way to see my purpose—as I oversaw the lives of others. At the end of my training at Wake Forest, I found the cards in my locker when I went to clean it out. They towered in the corners, one huge stack for those who had lived, and a shorter one for those who had died. I pulled out the survivor cards and shuffled through them. There was Teresa Martin. Names flashed into view on the other cards. A teacher with sepsis. The seventy-nine-year-old man with twin grand-daughters. Dr. Chin's grade-three epiglottis patient, too. I wondered where they all might be now. What they remembered about their stay and how often they thought of it. I imagined them and I felt gratitude, a healthy dose of pride that I'd had a modest hand in their outcome.

The smaller yet still-too-large pile of dead patient cards brought a different feeling, a lurch in the pit of my stomach about those who didn't make it. I gathered them up and held them. They seemed heavier than they should have, as if I were holding the full burden of death in my hands. I didn't want to look but then steeled myself and turned over the top card. Karras. I took a breath. She'd died so young, of acute myeloid leukemia. Her parents' names were on the card. I'd been close to Nancy and Rocky during their daughter's illness and death. They had gone to such extraordinary lengths to keep her alive; we all had. But the infection was too much for her body. I swallowed and put all the cards into my backpack. Maybe I'd read them later, when I was ready.

That evening, as soon as I returned home, I went straight to a file where I kept patients' correspondence and hunted for a letter. There it was, a little crumpled around the edges. I remembered reading it just after Karras had died. Rocky had written, "This morning Karras was taken off all attempts to save her. We were unable to perform the white blood cell transfer from Nancy to her, and the bacterial infection is too great to overcome. She is laboring to breathe, and we are making her comfortable. It is now a matter of how long she can make her body hold on. I can feel my heart bleed as I watch and wait for her passing. I am utterly devastated. There are no words to describe the depth of my excruciating sorrow."

I forced myself to digest this, his pain, Nancy's heartache. How close we came to saving their daughter but couldn't. It struck me then that the distance between the "living" and the "dead" stacks is extremely narrow, a hair, measured in minutes, perhaps, or fluid ounces. Yet it feels like a gaping void. The entire world. I knew it wasn't as simple an equation as this—that saving a life could be chalked up as success, while losing a patient meant we'd failed—yet that's how I felt. The critical care culture I'd immersed myself in promoted that belief.

It strikes me now how naive I was, not only by buying in, even partly, to that way of thinking. But by how simplistic was my division of patients into the living and the dead. The good outcomes and the bad. As if a myriad of nuances weren't in between.

I came of age as a doctor in the 1990s, trying as best I could to soak up everything happening in the frenetic world of the ICU. In medical school, I'd been enthralled by Guyton's classic physiology textbook on the workings of the human body, a rather dry tome to some, but it unleashed for me a song of admiration for the beauty and complexity of the mechanisms that make us living beings. The extraordinary communication and incessant coordination that have to take place between a vast array of systems just to keep us alive. As a new ICU doctor on rounds, the well-thumbed pages of Guyton would appear in my mind, the text clear and precise, the illustrations showing the way everything was supposed to function. In my ICU patients, everything was off. Their systems were disordered and leaning toward death.

At Wake Forest there were six different ICUs for adult admissions—medical, cardiovascular, surgical, burn, trauma, neuro—and we, in the medical ICU, prided ourselves that our patients were the sickest of the sick, often with multiple organ failure. I liked being one of the doctors whom others came to when things were looking desperate. We were the gatekeepers to the highest pinnacle of care in the hospital. When patients were ushered into our ICU, they were assured of the best that medicine could provide. Our unspoken understanding was that once patients came through those doors, we were the only thing standing between them and death. We were their best last chance. We blinded ourselves to the fact that one in three of our ventilated patients would not make it out alive, no matter how hard we tried.

We swept into action with our sophisticated machines, convinced that they would triumph. Ventilators, that evergreen symbol of life support, had advanced in astounding ways. The iron lungs that saved so many lives in the 1940s and '50s, and even the mechanical ventilators produced in the 1960s that had once been at the forefront of technology, looked laughable. By the 1990s, our ventilators had multiple dials with gauges and indicators allowing us to treat the lungs in increasingly detailed and tailored ways. It was as if we'd started using cameras with high-powered lenses, and we zoomed in on the lungs, focusing our care solely on them. These advances were one of the reasons I was drawn to specialize in pulmonary medicine. That, and the essential role that our lungs play in our survival. In essence, if we can't breathe, we die. It made sense to me that if I became a lung doctor, I'd be able to save more lives.

We take for granted our ability to breathe. We do it again and again, one breath after another, without thinking. Yet the lungs are incredibly complex, the respiratory system made up of so many different actors, structures, and functions. Cells with hairlike projections called cilia move fluid, goblet cells secrete mucus, and column-like cells line and protect. Our lungs have cells that are integral parts of our nervous system, lymphatic system, endocrine system, and our immune system. They contain cartilage, elastic tissue, connective tissue, muscle, and glands, and all of this gives rise to a system of airways that is fifteen hundred miles long—from New York City to Dallas—and filters every ounce of air entering the body. The lungs even have secret passages of air travel with evocative names such as pores of Kohn, canals of Lambert, and channels of Martin that bypass regular airways. There's a lung infection named Lady Windermere syndrome, named after the heroine of an Oscar Wilde comedy. I've always found all this fascinating. Our six liters of blood, traveling through the body at around four miles an hour, exchange carbon dioxide with oxygen from the seven liters of air we breathe per minute. In just one day, that's about ten thousand liters of air and eight thousand liters of blood coursing through sixty thousand miles of blood vessels, coming into contact with the surface of our air sacs, alveoli, that if spread out would be the size of a tennis court . . . all to maintain us as living, sentient beings.

My first clinical professor at Tulane, Dr. Watts Webb, brought the lungs to life for me. He always spoke of them with reverence and appreciation for the multiple roles they played in the body. I didn't know it at the time, but he had performed the first lung transplant in a human in 1963 along with Dr. James Hardy. In the clinic, Dr. Webb introduced us medical students to patients who complained of coughing up blood or having lost their wind, and in the operating room he showed us tumors, diseases of the airways, and scarring patterns from natural ailments and from smoking. There seemed to be so many ways that the lungs could be damaged. So many ways a doctor might be needed to fix their disorders and lean them back toward life.

The early ventilators with their simple "air in, air out" approach hadn't taken into account the elaborate nature of the lungs, in some ways hadn't respected it. As I continued my specialization in pulmonary medicine, I was still mesmerized reading Guyton's text, marveling at the orchestration of the respiratory system. I found a beauty in it, similar perhaps to how an artist admires a Rembrandt, the way the light, the colors, the brushstrokes all work together to create something more.

My aim with my patients was to get their broken systems back to functioning as they should, or as close to it as possible. The bright digits on the monitors and ventilator panels around the ICU bed told me the story of my patients' lungs, as well as the extent of the encroachment of illness. The numbers were usually devastating. In the ICU, the body is under assault, and my job was to find a way to manipulate the numbers through diagnosis and medicine, while dodging an onslaught of new threats. To make the numbers higher or lower as needed. And to do it all quickly. Stat. The trick was titration. One degree too much or too little of anything could send my patient over the edge and into the abyss. This was the part I loved. I kept my eyes on the machines, interpreting their messages, adjusting the ventilator settings, seeking the moment when the numbers would change for the better.

Sometimes the setup of my patients' breathing pattern—the speed of the delivery of their breaths by the ventilator and the correct dose of air—was particularly hard. Then, once I'd got it right, I'd sit at their bedside and marvel at the way their chest rose and fell, over and over. I'd watch the numbers improve as the tincture of time allowed the possibility of healing. I was surprised by how satisfying it was just to sit there and observe this unfolding in the midst of the busy ICU.

One of the first secrets of the trade we learn about as critical care doctors is positive end-expiratory pressure (PEEP). It's the kind of heaviness you feel pushing down into your chest when you blow up a balloon. For me, I always visualize Louis Armstrong, blowing on a trumpet with his puffed-up cheeks. I'd had New Orleans Jazz Fest prints of these scenes on my walls all through college and medical school, never realizing how important that image would become to me. That air pressing down into the lungs, deep into the alveoli, keeps millions of air sacs open and prevents their collapse. Turning a knob on the ventilator to supply PEEP is still one of the main treatments used in the ICU to save someone's life. We use it constantly to combat the desperately low oxygen levels in our COVID-19 pneumonia patients.

I'm always floored that this lifesaving intervention was discovered through sheer luck. In 1966, Dr. Michael Finnegan, a trainee in pulmonary medicine in Denver, Colorado, was working with the renowned Dr. Thomas Petty, the man who popularized portable and home oxygen therapy for patients with lung disease around the world. Their patient was dying of severe lung failure and low oxygen levels. This condition would be defined by Petty, the following year, as adult respiratory distress syndrome, later renamed acute respiratory distress syndrome (ARDS) after it was known to occur in children, too. As Finnegan stood at their patient's bedside trying to figure out a way to save her, he noticed a knob on the ventilator and turned it, sending more air pressing down into the lungs and keeping the air sacs open. Within minutes the patient's condition stabilized. An engineer had placed this knob on the machine in case it might be of help someday. Finnegan's curiosity turned into a lifesaving discovery about how best to treat ARDS, and PEEP became a cornerstone of the entire field of critical care.

From negative pressure to positive pressure to PEEP, progress continued in ventilation, enabling more lives to be saved as technology advanced, yet our sickest patients, those with extremely low oxygen levels, still continued to die. ICU doctors needed a different way of getting air into patients' lungs, and a new technique was developed to do just that. Inverse ratio ventilation (IRV), so called because it is the exact opposite of the way people breathe naturally, was the go-to method for our most tenuous patients when I trained as an intensivist. Humans breathe in and out at a ratio of around 1:3, meaning we exhale for three times longer than we inhale, but in IRV the patient is made to breathe at about a 2:1 ratio. If you try to do that now, taking a deep breath and holding it for two seconds, then blowing the air out in just one second and immediately taking another huge breath and holding it for two more seconds, you'll discover how uncomfortable it is. If you keep doing this, you'll find that after three or four cycles, your chest feels as if it were exploding. Now try to imagine being forced to breathe like that throughout today and tomorrow and beyond.

In my early years in the ICU, I kept many people alive on a ventilator using IRV, including some who would surely have moved to the shorter stack of index cards without it. I've seen the torture for the patients as they choke on air, panicked, fighting the ventilator. It's only possible to endure this treatment when deeply sedated and paralyzed, so, from the first days of using IRV, we critical care doctors gave our patients enormous doses of sedatives and paralytics around the clock to make sure they were unaware of what was happening to them. In this way, the machines breathed for these desperately ill patients while giving their bodies time to focus on getting better. Then, one or even two weeks later, we brought them out of their coma and transferred them to step-down care elsewhere in the hospital. Another life saved. How good it felt.

The pool of patients we saved grew even bigger. As we saw our success increase, we became used to seeing patients quiet on the ventilators as their lungs healed, and we applied this approach of intense sedation and paralysis to all our ventilated patients. It seemed to make sense.

• • •

The corner room in our ICU at Wake Forest had a view of towering oak trees and, in the distance, a gathering of houses, and whenever I had a second to spare, I'd contemplate the world beyond the window. My patients never looked outside. They were nearly always prostrate in their beds, tied down, and in comas. Rosa Allen was no different. For thirteen days, her face had pointed directly up at the bland tiled ceiling from a supine position, and her head had not moved more than twelve inches in any direction. I had never heard her voice and I'd never seen her awake. We referred to her, among the ICU team, as Bed Seven. Or, if we had more time, as Sepsis in Bed Seven. We rarely had more time though. She had come into the hospital to deliver a baby and, several days later, had contracted puerperal sepsis, a severe and life-threatening infection. The ob-gyn team had acted quickly and rushed her up to the ICU, where I'd intubated her, then hooked her up to a ventilator and the monitoring machines.

Dangling from the ceiling by tape and a piece of twine was a photo of her baby boy. The nurses had hung it there, motivated by Rosa's nine-year-old daughter, who wanted her mom to see a picture of her new baby the moment she woke up. That hadn't yet happened but I hoped it would soon. I had stopped Rosa's meds the day before. She had been on huge doses of pancuronium, midazolam, and fentanyl—the standard neuro-muscular blocker, benzodiazepine, and an opioid concoction that we gave to most of our patients. It worked to keep them calm. I sat and watched the rapid rise and slow fall of Rosa's chest, then looked up to see the picture twirl and sway as if the baby were dancing. I wondered whether Rosa would ever get to see it, much less the child himself. For a moment, I thought back on Sarah Bollich, my patient at Charity, who never left the ICU to see her baby again. We'd come a long way since then. The care was much better now. I hoped that it would work for Rosa.

Later in the day, I checked on her again, consulting the monitors over her bed. I sensed her eyes were open and turned to see her staring straight up, her eyes on the photo. Finally, she'd seen her baby. I placed my hand in hers, and she clutched it with stiff and swollen fingers and squinted up at me.

"She's awake," I said to Rosa's sister, Harriet, who'd just arrived in the room. Her face lit up, tears in her eyes.

Rosa squirmed in the bed, rolling her eyes back to the picture.

"That's your baby, Mrs. Allen." I was smiling now.

Rosa just stared at me, her eyes wide with shock.

"He's yours. You held him in your arms and named him."

"Yes, you did," said Harriet, grinning.

But Rosa shook her head. I handed her a white board and a pen. "Not my baby," she scribbled. Then again, "Not my baby." She sighed and closed her eyes.

I felt bewildered, even irritated. I was trying to save a mother for her son. I turned to Harriet, asking, "How can you forget having a baby?"

She shook her head, her mouth squeezed shut, as if she were trying to keep her feelings inside. She sat down in the brown vinyl hospital chair at her sister's side and hunched forward, her hands clasped as if in prayer. "Maybe she needs more time."

I nodded. Maybe Rosa's body wasn't ready to be awake yet. I turned up the drip rate on the sedatives, then spoke to her nurse. "Let's start her on five milligrams of intravenous haloperidol every six hours." I thought the antipsychotic would help with Rosa's confusion. Clearly she had ICU psychosis, a common side effect of being in the ICU. I stood awhile and watched as her face relaxed. She was unconscious again. I hoped that somewhere in the fog of her dreams, she would see her little boy and recognize him as her own.

Two weeks later, I watched twilight slipping in through the windows, dusting the tops of the oak trees purple. I had just wished Rosa well as she and her new son headed home. She had finally accepted that the baby was hers and had spent long hours in our step-down unit, gazing into his eyes. I was glad that she had survived against the odds and would get to see her family grow. That we had moved forward since Sarah Bollich's death at Charity. My shift was over and I turned to leave, walking through the twenty-five-bed ICU. My patients—Cirrhosis in Bed Five, Heart Failure in Nine, ARDS in Twelve, among others—were all silent, attached to ventilators keeping death at bay, alarms and monitors watching over them. All was as it should have been. As I'd been taught. Yet, in the back of my mind I sensed that something wasn't right. Was this the best way to practice medicine?

Chapter 4

The World of Transplant Medicine— Harvesting the Right Path Forward

I had gone from being ignorant of being ignorant to being aware of being aware.

—Maya Angelou, *I Know Why the Caged Bird Sings*

"**WHAT I SEE THESE** days are paralyzed, sedated patients, lying without motion, appearing to be dead, except for the monitors that tell me otherwise." I couldn't get this quote out of my head. It had appeared in the medical journal *Chest* in an explosive editorial written by the celebrated Dr. Thomas Petty about what he saw as a crisis in critical care. This was 1998. Every day, as I made rounds in the ICU, his words resonated in my mind. Nearly all my critically ill patients were exactly as he described, unconscious and paralyzed in their beds. Some had been like that for endless days. Petty had gone on to say that in the past, patients on ventilators were rarely paralyzed and were only given morphine or occasional low doses of sedatives. This seemed astonishing to me. Some of my colleagues considered his arguments for a return to less sedation and an increased focus on "the basic principles of human caring" as the thoughts of a Luddite who didn't know anything about the latest ventilators, but his words struck a chord with me. I had a feeling that we should be handling our patients in a very different way.

On an average day, five to eight patients were admitted to my care, most of whom either came in on a ventilator or ended up on one. I'd started to feel unsettled seeing them lying there, tethered to their machines, stuck in suspended animation. It seemed that the sense of urgency we all felt when a patient was admitted, that shot of adrenaline that flared as we actively sought to save a life, dissipated once the ventilator was in place. It was as if we handed over care of our patients to the machines while we went off and admitted, intubated, sedated, and paralyzed the next one. My noble mission of saving lives had turned into a conveyor belt of care.

What's more, Dr. Petty, in his article, listed medical complications that often arose when a patient was immobilized: nerve damage, muscle weakness, serious infections, and a kind of foggy thinking known as intensive care delirium. As I read through his list, I felt a creeping chill rise up my spine. It was eerily similar to the catalog of complaints that Teresa Martin's mother had detailed when they returned to my clinic weeks after she was discharged from the ICU. Petty called for less sedation and paralysis, for more sitting at our patients' bedsides. I didn't disagree. I just wasn't sure how to make it happen in the ICU, whether it was even possible.

• • •

Several months before the publication of Petty's editorial, I had finished training in lung transplantation at Barnes-Jewish Hospital in St. Louis, Missouri, and headed back to Wake Forest, where the Chief of Medicine, Dr. William Hazzard, had hired me as the medical director of a brand-new heart-and-lung-transplant program. Dr. Hazzard, one of the founding fathers of geriatric medicine, had become my mentor the year before. I had shared an office wall with him, soaking up his knowledge and his generosity in communicating it to me. He had supported my move into the world of transplant, agreeing that it was a natural extension of critical care. It seemed visionary to me, so innovative in the way it pushed at the bounds of medicine. The idea of taking patients who lived in the ever-lengthening shadow of death and bringing them back into the light of life by transplantation was hard to resist, as was the thought of manipulating the immune system into accepting another person's lung. I was sure that constant exposure to the contrast of life and death would be exhilarating yet sobering. Awe-inspiring in the actual sense of the word. What I didn't expect was that I'd leave with a completely new way of seeing critical care.

In going into transplant, a part of me felt I was following in the footsteps of my Tulane professor Dr. Watts Webb, though the field had greatly evolved since his pioneering work in the early 1960s. Curious about his involvement in the first lung transplant on June 11, 1963, I read up on the history and was surprised to learn, with some digging, that the patient, John Russell, was a hospitalized prison inmate with lung cancer who had agreed to undergo the procedure as a last resort. This information tended to be missing from most accounts, as was the fact that Mississippi state government authorities suggested "a very favorable attitude" would be taken toward the prisoner if he helped advance science in this manner. While the first lung transplant was undoubtedly a monumental milestone in medical history, I was struck by the tidy emphasis, in the official record, on the progress of critical care, not the patient caught up in its wake.

Something else drew my attention while I read. Just past midnight, as this first lung transplant patient lay in recovery after the grueling surgery, a thirty-seven-year-old man took his last breath in the same hospital's emergency room. A white supremacist had shot the great American civil rights leader Medgar Evers with a rifle at close range. The lifesaving triumph of the transplant juxtaposed with this devastating death shook me. It seemed significant that while Evers's assassination dominated headlines the next day, and news of the transplant was just a small article in the corner, over time the march of medical progress became the important event of that night. This first human lung transplant in small-town Mississippi caught the world's attention and advanced the entire field of organ transplantation. In contrast, the outrage expressed over Evers's death did not lead to immediate progress in the fight against racism, and the struggle for civil rights forged on. It seemed that two pieces of history moved in opposite directions under the same roof, the human players left in the wake, and social injustices papered over.

Barnes-Jewish was the mecca for the rapidly advancing field of transplant medicine, and I had the honor of training with Dr. Bert Trulock, then the leading transplant pulmonologist in the country. As a visiting doctor, I accompanied him as he cared for his patients, who were all in the end stages of lung disease and lived with a chronic feeling of suffocation—and lingering hope that they'd make it off the organ waiting list in time. I was struck by how well Dr. Trulock knew them all, joking about their favorite sports teams, inquiring about their partner's health, and knowing which of their children was about to graduate high school. As I spent more time there, I, too, got to know his patients.

An enormous amount of screening goes on before someone is placed on the organ transplant waiting list. Once we had completed all the medical testing and determined that our patients' only health problem was severly failing lungs, we would ask them about themselves. Not just their medical history, though that was important, but also personality details, their employment information, their living situation, their family support system, all to see whether they and their caregivers would be a good fit for the rigors of life as an organ transplant recipient. We often told patients that they would be trading one set of problems for another. After transplant they would have to take twenty to thirty pills a day for the rest of their lives to ward off rejection of the new lung. This would suppress their immune system, which would leave them vulnerable to infection. We needed to be sure that a loved one would be available and willing to help with their care. As I listened, I started to see beyond the here and now of my hospital office where they were our patients, and out into the worlds they had created where they worked and loved and dreamed. Fragile lives made vulnerable by destructive diseases that left them chronically and critically ill.

There was the woman in her sixties, a never-smoker, who came in with persistent wheezing, shortness of breath, and recurrent infections. During her two-hour patient history, she told us how her daily walk with Bobby, her spaniel mix, had shortened from a two-mile loop through grassy fields to a slow shuffle to the end of her driveway. Even that left her gasping. Laboratory testing confirmed our outlandish suspicion that she had previously undiagnosed cystic fibrosis—which is usually diagnosed during childhood—and we put her on the list for the double-lung transplant that would open up her life again.

Another patient had developed severe scarring in both his lungs that made a trip to the mailbox an arduous undertaking, one he could manage only once or twice a week. During his family history, he regaled us with stories of his relatives, and we noted curious similarities between his symptoms and theirs. Over time I understood his disease to be an inheritable form of pulmonary fibrosis and experienced the joy of seeing him through a single-lung transplant and back into his life. Not only did his new lung enable him to walk much farther than to his mailbox, it also, as he told us with some glee, allowed him to outlive all his relatives.

I listened to the stories told by Trulock's patients and realized how little thought I'd given to the lives my ICU patients led beyond the confines of my care. We doctors are supposed to ask our patients questions about themselves as part of the standard complete history and physical, but in critical care we didn't always consider it relevant. Often it wasn't practical, as our patients' lives were in the balance and speed was of the essence. We focused on the physical, the body itself. Then we zoomed in even more, homing in on a specific body part. An organ. For me, my ICU patients were usually reduced to a lung.

One could argue that the earliest form of medical technology was the stethoscope, invented in 1816 in France by Dr. René Laënnec. Until then, physicians gained knowledge about a patient's illness from a visual inspection of the body and from the patient's story about his illness. But, beginning with Laënnec's first "wooden tube" stethoscope, doctors subtly started to shift focus to information conveyed by their newly invented tools. As medical advances continued, patients' voices became increasingly stripped from their stories. Nowhere was this truer than with deeply sedated patients on mechanical ventilators. I saw that, in many ways, transplant candidates were their polar opposite, serving as their own advocates and divulging their entire human story to gain the support of a team and receive a lifesaving organ.

I found it interesting that in transplant, the failing organ was our starting point. From there we pulled back to see the patient as a person. Trulock and I met with each patient many times over the course of their illness: during the months while they waited for an organ, seeing them grow sicker and weaker, life and hope ebbing out of them. We'd meet again before surgery when finally a suitable lung was available, and then afterward, seeing them back at the clinic every month to adjust their medications and manage their immunosuppression and infection risks. I would hear about the new milestones in their lives. The first time they drove again or went out to eat or held their grandchild. The simple stuff of life. I liked the intensity of these interactions with my transplant patients.

In contrast, I saw my contact with my ICU patients as akin to that of the transplant surgeons who sewed in the new organs. For some surgeons, the longest time they spent with the transplant patients was when they operated on them. Then they sent them home with new lungs, their life saved, with most of the day-to-day care falling back to Trulock and me. I didn't want to be that kind of physician anymore.

• • •

When I returned to North Carolina, I carried with me the hope that I could bring what I'd learned at Barnes-Jewish to my doctoring at the new heart-and-lung-transplant clinic. My first patient, a young man about my age, came down from Cobb Holler in the foothills of the Blue Ridge Mountains to see me about a new heart and lungs. I could have guessed this even if he hadn't told me, as he was completely blue. As Marcus Cobb walked into my examining room with his wife and two small children, he smiled as if he had some secret test for me.

His brown eyes were large, pleading, but I didn't return his gaze. I was drawn to his skin. It was the color of faded denim, his lips dark purple like a bruise. We call this cyanosis, and with his degree of "blueness," I could tell that more than a third of his hemoglobin was coursing through his body without any oxygen. Marcus had Eisenmenger's syndrome. The right side of his heart was too big and was forcing used blood from his veins over to the left side of his heart and out to his body without first going through the lungs to pick up oxygen. My eyes moved to his chest.

A burly guy, he started out a little confrontational. "Listen, Dr. Ely." I looked up. "I'm blue because I was born with holes in my heart, and I've had one foot in a casket since I was a little boy," he said with a Southern twang. "Many all-knowing doctors have told me I'm about to die. They've all been wrong so far, but now at thirty-two, Danita and I are wondering?"

Then they both just looked at me. Danita seemed hopeful, as if I could cure her husband with a wave of my hand. Marcus's presence in my clinic was extraordinary. Normally, when someone's blood oxygen levels go below 90 percent in the ICU, we begin to intervene. Yet there was Marcus, sitting in front of me with oxygen levels that must have been around 65 percent. And he had been living that way for the past three decades. I didn't know what to say. Who was I to decide when it would be time to cut his chest open, remove his heart and lungs, and sew in someone else's? I knew that with transplant, timing is everything, and it's imperative to get it right. You want to put it off until the last minute. As soon as new organs are placed, the immune system's rejection clock starts its countdown. While this can be slowed, it can't be stopped entirely. New organs come with their own built-in death sentence. But you also can't wait too long, or the person will die on the wait list.

As I considered all this, I started to feel uncomfortable. Danita and the children needed Marcus to be alive and well, and they had come to me for help. They had placed all their hopes in my hands, and I was overwhelmed. I didn't have Trulock to turn to. Marcus was my responsibility alone, and he sat waiting for my answer. I began to flush and perspire, asking questions as best I could and learning about his life, his work designing security systems, the couple's challenges, their children, Ariel and Ty, and there were Jay, Patrick, and Lacey, too, from Marcus's previous marriage. My questions weren't helping me. They were only making his life larger. More precious. I was a father now to three young daughters, and their sweet faces flashed into my mind. I felt huge beads of sweat forming on my forehead then rolling down my cheeks and landing on papers on my desk. I tried to act as if everything were fine, but I could feel my face burning. Marcus was talking about Ariel's Barbie collection.

I excused myself and slipped into the nearest bathroom, closed the door, and stared at the tiled wall. Taking off my white coat, I saw that my light blue shirt was drenched through with sweat. I tried to work out what was wrong. I had all the technical training I needed to be a good doctor to Marcus: four years of medical school, three years as a resident, one as chief resident, three years specializing in critical care and the lungs, and finally my lung transplant fellowship in St. Louis. I'd treated critically ill patients for years in the ICU, so that wasn't new, either. But seeing Marcus in front of me, seriously ill, deeply invested in his life, human, awake, and my responsibility alone—that was weighty.

I slinked back into the examining room, head low, took out my stethoscope, and completed a cursory physical examination. I explained to Marcus how to adjust his fluid pills, told them I'd like to see them again in a couple of months, that they should be in touch if things started to worsen. Then they were gone. I was convinced I'd been added to their list of failed doctors and never expected to see either of them again.

• • •

The experience with Marcus Cobb created a crisis of confidence in me. I'd felt so comfortable in transplant with the team at Barnes-Jewish, but back at Wake Forest I felt alone and unsure. I wanted to be in the trenches with my patients but wasn't convinced I was the right person to be running a new program, now that I'd seen how I handled the responsibility of meeting my patients in their lives.

I remembered the ideals I'd had in medical school, my friend Dr. Darin Portnoy and I on the roof at Charity, declaring a commitment to making a difference for the unheard. He was already leading a tuberculosis-control program with Médecins Sans Frontières in Uzbekistan. I, on the other hand, had failed with Marcus, just one patient. He'd come to me, and I'd sent him away. Most of my other patients were on ventilators, dead to the world for all intents and purposes. I certainly wasn't speaking up for them—I barely knew their names. I seemed to have lost a fundamental part of myself, of the doctor I'd wanted to be, now that I was a specialist in critical care.

I'd read F. Scott Fitzgerald in college. In his first novel, *This Side of Paradise*, the directionless Amory Blaine had especially resonated with me. I'd been fascinated by Blaine precisely because of his aimlessness, which was so alien to me. But now I found myself identifying with him as I endeavored to find my way. I'd finally finished my medical training, which I'd pursued with a laser focus, and should have been striding into the future. Yet I muddled forward. Fitzgerald's description of Blaine ran through my mind: "It was always the becoming he dreamed of, never the being."

A couple of years earlier, I'd published my chief-resident research project in the *New England Journal of Medicine*. I had felt excitement and shock that my first paper was well received, and that finally the elite club of critical care had admitted me into its ranks. The study investigated how to wean patients from the ventilator using what quickly became known as spontaneous breathing trials (SBTs), and built on work by Dr. Martin Tobin from Chicago and a famous Spanish lung doctor, Andrés Esteban. During my training, I'd been struck by the way every doctor seemed to have a completely different approach to deciding when patients were ready to come off a ventilator. One might turn the breathing rate down gradually from eighteen breaths a minute to fourteen and then ten over many hours of weaning, while another might allow patients themselves to determine the number of breaths, but provide less assistance from the ventilator at each breath. Whatever the method, most of the weaning approaches appeared arbitrary, and none of them seemed especially scientific about when to initiate the process.

My study focused on the creation of a weaning standard, one that respiratory therapists and nurses as well as doctors could use. In this way, the patient could continue to advance even if the doctor was elsewhere. The idea was simply to take all ventilated patients off the ventilator for a short time each day, to see if they were ready to breathe unassisted. This was deemed radical by doctors, who largely assumed that a rapid removal of life support would create havoc. They felt it could cause heart attacks or strokes in a person so critically ill, but I had done my homework. I had a hunch but didn't initially know what kind of results to expect. I was astonished when we proved in our study of three hundred patients with respiratory failure over one year that this simple standardization allowed us to remove patients from the ventilator a full two days earlier, cut medical complications in half, and save $5,000 per patient in hospital costs. It turned out that the decades-old practice of removing the ventilator slowly could be safely accelerated. When patients were ready to breathe on their own, they could be liberated, not weaned. It felt like a victory.

Yet, for all the excitement caused by the paper, it didn't seem to move the needle much. My ventilated patients were still sedated and paralyzed for days on end. I felt stuck. My job was to stare at monitors and machines, and for all my love of Guyton and physiology, something important was missing.

• • •

Soon after, in the summer of 1998, my family and I moved to Nashville, Tennessee, so that Kim could pursue further training as a surgical pathology fellow at Vanderbilt University. I was still unsure what path I was on and was relieved to follow Kim, who knew what she was doing. Once we'd settled in, I was hired to be the co–medical director of the lung transplant program there, and I started to enjoy my work in the clinic. It felt familiar, much the same as I'd been doing with Trulock at Barnes-Jewish, collaborating with a team, evaluating patients, completing their transplant workup, organizing their transplant listing, and seeing them through to the other side of their new existence. Many of them told me, "You know, Doc, every day is a gift day." I was getting better with the patient interactions, in part because I knew I was backed by a long-established transplant center.

One afternoon, I sauntered into a clinic room to see a new patient for a heart-lung transplant evaluation. The first thing I saw was blue skin, then purple lips, and next the burdened faces of Marcus and Danita. They had tracked me down and driven six hours to see me. Marcus had deteriorated badly, and his boggy, fluid-filled ankles, heart gallop, and crackly lung sounds told the tale. I knew the timing was now right. Marcus needed a heart and two lungs, and quickly, or he was not long for this world.

After I had completed the history and medical testing, I had a question for them. "Why in the world would you want to see me again after I made such a fool of myself when we first met?" In her thick Southern drawl, Danita said, "When we left you that day, we knew you realized that you didn't have all the answers. That's why we said to each other that you were going to be our doctor. So here we are."

Marcus Cobb became my patient, and I placed him on the list for new organs. The waiting began. He and Danita packed their suitcases, and a call was made to a charter flight company so that when the time came, if it did, they would be ready to leave at a moment's notice. His heart and lungs continued to decline. But then late one night, after about a month of waiting, I received a call from a Tennessee organ-sharing organization. They had donor organs for Marcus. I called the Cobbs' home, and when I gave him the news, I heard his tired voice quicken with hope. "Honey, get the bags," he said. "We're going to Nashville."

Along with my happiness for Marcus, I felt the underlying heaviness that always accompanies these calls, the knowledge that, somewhere, someone else had to die to gift these organs. That even now the person's loved ones would be grieving. I hung up the phone, and in the quiet of my house, my family safe and sleeping, I sat alone with thoughts of gratitude. Thankful for the courage of strangers.

The next day at Vanderbilt, I waited. Finally, the surgeon came out of the operating room, looking haggard after the nine-hour surgery, and told me he had struggled with blood vessels as thick as ropes that had developed in Marcus's chest over his life. But the operation was a success. Marcus was wheeled into the ICU on a gurney, and I saw immediately that he was no longer blue. We set him up with everything we could offer to support his new organs and his recovering body.

Over the next few days, I stayed at his bedside, overseeing the monitors, adjusting his blood pressure medications, his ventilator, the dosage of sedatives, antibiotics, and immune-suppressing medications.

Everything needed to be titrated exactly. This was why I'd trained in transplant, this kind of shoot-for-the-moon medicine, but now it was completely different. I found myself looking at Marcus's face as he lay there, watching as he pulled every deep-drawn breath into his new lungs, and pondering the mystery of his flickering life. I knew him intimately. Not the notes-scribbled-on-an-index-card kind of knowing; much deeper than that. I knew his family, too, and they were by my side, constantly, holding Marcus's hand and talking to him, cheering him on. It struck me that they were life support for him, too. For once, I wasn't thinking just about Marcus's lungs or heart. I finally had the whole person in my scope.

• • •

I believe Marcus was the first patient whom I truly saw as a whole person. I hadn't understood that I could enter my patients' lives to the degree I did with him and his family, and that doing so would make me a better doctor. During my months of aimlessness, I had expanded my reading, trying to gain some insight and self-knowledge. After Marcus's transplant I started to connect the dots. I had read Ignatius of Loyola's *Spiritual Exercises*, written in the 1500s, in which he teaches about our frequent failure as humans to attain fullness in relationships, and I began to understand the impact of my failings on my patients. I had always cared for them and wanted to do my best for them as their doctor, but I was treating them as inanimate objects, in what philosopher Martin Buber describes as an "I-it" relationship. I had collected data and analyzed and classified them, seeing my patients as a set of organs to fix and a list of problems to solve. I had read and recommended Samuel Shem's novel *The House of God*, about an overworked intern learning the ropes in a hospital. Shem's narrator, while hilariously entertaining, depersonalized patients, using disparaging terms such as *Gomer* (Get Out of My Emergency Room). I saw now that I, too, had showed callous disregard for some of my patients. I had thought it innocuous to use Gallbladder in Room 557 to consolidate both person and diagnosis, without digging any deeper. I wasn't seeing my patients as fully human. Did they know?

Now, looking back, I suspect many did. As a medical student, and during my training, I was often taught to keep a professional sense of reserve and mental distance from patients, that getting to know them too well would backfire and cause me stress if they should die. When I graduated from Tulane Medical School in 1989, my mom had given me a leatherbound copy of Dr. William Osler's "Aequanimitas," his famous address delivered to new doctors at the Pennsylvania School of Medicine exactly one hundred years earlier. Osler's words, advice derived from Aristotle, became a touchstone for me: "Deep voice, slow speech, tight compartments, with the mind directed intensely on the subject at hand." I carried the quote with me every day on a handwritten card in the pocket of my white coat, as if doing so would allow me to connect directly to them both. I had used equanimity many times as a tool to pause, pull back, and process. To maintain balance and composure. Now I wondered if I had withdrawn my feelings, too.

But, finally, with Marcus, I experienced what Buber calls an "I-Thou" encounter, meeting him fully within his life. I'd been reluctant and it had taken me a long time, but he and Danita had persisted. I was so glad that they did. Thanks to them, I was finding my way forward as a doctor again.

Marcus's heart-lung transplantation became the gift he'd dreamed of, not only giving him more time with Danita and his children, but also the opportunity to embrace activities he'd only imagined in the past. Going for long sunset hikes in the Blue Ridge Mountains, even parachuting from helicopters. He grabbed at life with both hands. But during our monthly and, later, quarterly clinic visits, I noted with a smile that the activities that seemed to give him the most pleasure in his new life were the smaller things, such as simply throwing a football with his kids.

• • •

As we knew would happen, all good things fade, and this is most certainly true for the tenure of organs at the whim of a stubborn immune system. Several years later, I was about to give a lecture to a few hundred physicians at a medical conference in San Diego when my phone rang. It was Danita: "Marcus is dying. He's asking for you." Without hesitation, I apologized to the meeting organizers and rushed to the airport to catch a plane home. It was a particularly clear day, and from my window seat, I watched the canyons and lakes pass beneath us, praying all the while that I'd get there in time.

In the cab from the Nashville airport, on my way to Vanderbilt, I called Danita to ask for the room number. "It's number five on the eighth floor . . . but hurry." At the hospital, I sped to the elevators and shot out into the hallway. As I rounded the corner, through an open door I saw a crowd. I slipped into a nearly complete circle of about seven others. They'd been waiting for me. I put my hand on Marcus's shoulder, looked him in the eyes, and talked directly to him. He was the only person in the world who mattered at that moment. It had become second nature to me by then. He looked up at me and I whispered, "Thank you." Then Marcus died.

• • •

After Marcus, I found a kind of fulfillment with the transplant patients in my care. I often felt humility around them, seeing the courage it took them to face each day with chronic illness, and observing their zest for life post-transplant, knowing they lived on borrowed time. For them, their illness and treatment were so inextricably bound with their life that it was impossible to separate the two.

I met a man with a chronic lung condition named Danny West. He was six feet tall and lanky and always stood slightly crooked, with one knee bent. Danny had an ease about him that made me relax, and a magnificently bushy handlebar mustache that bounced up and down when he laughed. His illness meant that I saw him often, and he drew me in. I allowed myself to flow into the covenant of our friendship in a way I would have considered reckless even just one year earlier. Maybe it made me vulnerable, but it felt right and true.

One spring day, Danny accompanied me to the medical school, where I was teaching a hundred budding doctors about the lung sounds they might hear through a stethoscope during a patient's physical examination. Danny, who had one healthy transplanted lung, and one old, scarred lung, was a good candidate for this demonstration. The students would hear the free flow of air on one side of his chest and the crackling cacophony of sputtering air on the other. A year earlier I had taught the same lecture and followed my usual practice of asking for a student volunteer to be examined in front of the class. A young woman had stood up and made her way down the stairs to the bottom of the large amphitheater. There, she took off her blouse, showing her leopard-skin bra, and the entire class roared with laughter. This year Danny was my ace-in-the-hole substitute to avoid such a fiasco. I explained to the class what we were about to embark on and asked Danny to remove his shirt so I could examine him. I turned away to grab my stethoscope and was startled to hear a wave of thunderous applause and howling laughter throughout the cavernous hall. Turning around, I saw Danny grinning mischievously at me, proudly sporting a leopard-skin bra.

Even later, when that old rotten lung became the source of a fatal cancer that spread to his brain, Danny never lost his sense of humor. I went to see him in the oncology clinic toward the end, and he poked fun at himself. I knew it would be the last time I would ever see him. It wouldn't be the last time he made me laugh, though. That happened at his funeral, where I'd been asked to speak by his wife, Becky. Danny had left me a framed picture of us from the day with the medical students and a poem he'd written himself, and they made me laugh through tears. He'd invited me to be a part of his life beyond the hospital and all the way through to his death. And I had accepted.

. . .

My transplant patients awoke something in me—a need for more humanity in doctoring—and I wanted to bring it to my ventilated patients in the ICU. I just wasn't sure how to embrace it in the world of critical care. I knew I needed to lift my eyes from the monitors to my patients' faces, and to pull my gaze back from their broken lungs to see them as people, dislocated from their lives and eager to return. But how could I do that when they were rushed to me in medical emergencies, sedated and paralyzed, without agency or voice?

As I was trying to work out how to combine the technology-bound world of the ICU with the humanism of transplant, I was invited to a talk in Nashville, given by Dr. Thomas Petty himself. It was just a couple of years after his editorial had appeared in *Chest*. While he may have riled up some in the critical care community, he was still revered and respected for the many contributions he'd made to the field. I was excited to be in his presence and to hear what he might say. The talk took place at a local restaurant called F. Scott's (which seemed especially fitting to me, even though I was no longer channeling Amory Blaine). After Dr. Petty finished speaking about patients living with chronic respiratory illnesses, I had an epiphany. I realized these patients had frequent contact with their doctor. I had only been thinking about my patients within the bounds of the ICU, but what about after they left my care?

When they were discharged home. I didn't even know where they went for ongoing care when they needed it. I wondered if I should be seeing them back at my clinic for monthly or quarterly follow-ups, as I did with the transplant patients. Around me everyone was applauding, and I joined in, feeling inspired. I went up to Petty with a well-worn copy of his editorial in hand. We looked together at his closing paragraph, at his call for more humanity in medicine.

I asked him, "What do you think we should do?"

He wrinkled his eyebrows. "You want the solution to the problem?" He peered at me, his bow tie a little to one side. "I honestly still don't know," he quipped softly, "but maybe you can help figure it out."

Chapter 5

Delirium Disaster—An Invisible Calamity for Patients and Families

A long habit of not thinking a thing wrong gives it a superficial appearance of being right.

—Thomas Paine, *Common Sense*

DURING THE COVID-19 PANDEMIC, Ray Fugate sat lopsided, legs askew, in his bedside chair. His secretion-streaked breathing tube, sticking a few inches out of his mouth and connected to the ventilator on his left, whizzed 380 ml breaths into him eighteen to twenty-four times a minute, just the right calibration. Sunshine flooded through the large window and highlighted his short reddish-brown hair, which stood straight up in the back, giving him a boyish appearance. He waved a small whiteboard at me, looking frustrated. This is the way he communicated with us, and I could see the big red words he'd written in marker: "Let me go see Shelley." His wife of thirty years. He had been in the ICU for two weeks, while the coronavirus destroyed the lining of his fifty-one-year-old lungs. On rounds that morning, I had heard the familiar snap, crackle, and pop of Rice Krispies across the front and back of his chest. He was struggling with deadly COVID pneumonia. Now Ray was writing all over his whiteboard, and when he held it up again, the words didn't make any sense. It was just a scribble of red ink. As much as his lungs were burdened by disease, his brain had it even worse. He had delirium. It was a devastating presence with this virus, and an ICU stay exacerbated the effects, especially when we couldn't have family at the bedside. Ray needed Shelley, his childhood sweetheart.

The next day, his delirium lifted and he improved enough for us to remove the ventilator and try less aggressive ways of delivering oxygen. This also meant he and Shelley could talk on the phone. Unfortunately, as he spoke, he spiraled down into delirium again and his oxygen levels dropped. I heard him yelling, "Shelley, come and get me now, they're trying to kill me. Shelley, they won't let me leave. They're holding me against my will. Shelley, I have to get out of here." It was heartrending to listen to his rants, to know the fear he felt was real, and especially to know that we were likely to have to hook him up to the ventilator again and take away his voice.

I geared up, pulling on my personal protective clothing and my electronically powered air purifying respirator, or PAPR, which protects me against airborne particles, and strode into his room, Darth Vader in white. I knelt by his chair and held his hands, pointed at the clock, and told him again, "Mr. Fugate, I'm so glad you are up and out of bed, and I'm sorry you are confused. I just spoke with Shelley, and she'll be here in two hours, at one p.m., to talk to you on the phone out there in the hall through the glass wall of your room. Most importantly, she said to tell you she loves you!"

It astonishes me now that we never used to pay attention to delirium as a meaningful medical injury in our critical care patients. We noticed it only because it inconvenienced us as physicians, then we dismissed it as a completely normal, to-be-expected side effect of serious illness and treatment in an ICU. It took a long time before we realized that it could be harmful to our patients in many ways.

• • •

As a young doctor in late 1999, buoyed by a growing confidence in my ability to connect more with my patients and a desire to know them better, I started to follow them to the non-ICU-floor beds where they were transferred once they were stable enough. I'd stop by to see how they were doing. It felt strange at first, as if I were trespassing, and I half expected someone to send me back to my own floor. The patients weren't mine anymore, after all. They were under other doctors' care now.

I stood at the end of the bed and introduced myself to them, to their loved ones, and, if invited, pulled up a chair. I made a point of using their names. "Hello, Mr. Ramirez, I'm Dr. Ely from upstairs, and I'm just here to see how you're feeling today." Something about this transaction, away from my machines, was very simple. Sometimes I heard the patient's voice clearly for the first time or saw their eyes shine with hope, not fear. In the ICU, I mostly saw the whites of patients' eyes, panic welling up, especially if a breathing tube prevented them from speaking. On the non-ICU wards, I noticed that some patients were calmer as they moved beyond their time on life support. There they started to think about the future, going home.

But in other patients, I saw fear and uncertainty. As if they had been pushed into a strange land and were unable to get their bearings. These patients were especially glad to see me. They knew I understood what they had just been through. I was a familiar presence in a disorienting place.

In the beginning, I stayed just a minute or two, but then as I grew into this new role, I lingered, listening to families reunite and reconnect on the other side of critical illness. A surprising theme began to stand out. The patients and their families told completely different narratives about the patient's stay in the ICU. Often a patient had little idea that she had been so seriously ill, had a tenuous understanding of procedures undergone, and remembered almost nothing about her loved ones' visits or interactions she'd had with them. In addition, she seemed to have spent her entire time on the ventilator in a terrifyingly realistic alternate universe. I heard one patient describe an attack by a mob of green aliens; another recounted a story about being swarmed by snakes; and yet another said he was constantly being pushed down a long, dark tunnel. I listened to story after story with a sense of growing comprehension and alarm. We had thought our ventilated patients were sleeping, protected by sedatives, paralytics, and pain medication from the intense discomfort caused by life-support machines. But clearly, they were not serenely dreaming. They were delirious, afraid and confused. When family members turned to me, looking for help in how to respond, I was unsure. Should they dismiss the stories and say that they weren't real, or should they acknowledge them, suggest they were hallucinations and delusions? Neither response seemed especially reassuring to the patient.

I started to think about these stories all the time, why the patients were experiencing delirium and why I hadn't fully realized how common it was. Our response to delirium was intravenous haloperidol, the primary drug used to manage psychosis since the 1950s and then the go-to treatment for many neurological conditions. It was first used for delirium in critically ill patients in 1973 when Dr. Edwin "Ned" Cassem, a much-respected cigar-smoking Jesuit-priest doctor and former chief of psychiatry at Massachusetts General Hospital, needed a safe way to calm an agitated patient who was critically ill with cardiogenic shock. Since then it had become standard practice around the world.

I wondered if we should be doing more. Back in the ICU, I began to look for signs of delirium, and I soon started to see that it was widespread among my ventilated patients. As the iconic Dr. William Osler once said, "Listen to your patient, he is telling you the diagnosis." I hadn't been listening—or looking—hard enough, or maybe not at all. I had been too confident in my ability to control everyone's passage through illness.

The first patients who told me through their behavior that they had delirium were those who railed against restraints and thrashed in their beds. When they woke up from sedation, they thought the nurses were poisoning them, or their families were scheming against them. I had never considered that they might be hallucinating and seeing terrible things even as I stood in front of them. Maybe they thought I was there to harm them. In the past, I had dismissed this as ICU psychosis, as a normal and benign response to being in the ICU. I had just thought these patients were angry about being strapped down, bothered by the noise or the lack of sleep, and I had felt frustrated that they were getting in the way of my care of them. Their lack of logic had bothered me, too. If they were upset about being tied down at the wrists, the way to persuade staff to remove the restraints was not by becoming violent. Now I saw how wrong I had been. Their brains weren't functioning properly, and they needed extra care. I just wasn't sure what that meant exactly, so I upped the doses of sedatives and antipsychotics to calm them down and to appease the stressed nurses and frightened families.

I started listening to my patients' loved ones, too, when they visited the ICU and said, "He's just not himself" or "She's not making any sense." They didn't know it, but they were alerting me to a quiet type of delirium that was easy to overlook. Previously, I had disregarded this fuzzy thinking as a normal by-product of critical illness. But I started to pay attention. If a patient woke up peacefully from sedation and answered questions with nods and smiles, but didn't recognize me as her doctor ten minutes after I had stopped by her bedside, I now saw it as a sign that something was off. On rounds, I made a point of asking the nurses to look out for confusion as a possible symptom of delirium.

"There you go again, Dr. Ely. The patient just has ICU psychosis. Everyone gets that, and it's not a big deal. It'll be gone before he goes home."

No one else seemed worried about delirium in the ICU. I'd never heard a single lecture or even a short teaching session about ICU delirium in all my years of training. I was aware of the classic work on delirium by Drs. George Engel and John Romano from the *Journal of Neuropsy-*

chiatry in 1959, but could find no similar work in the area of critical illness. Using an electroencephalogram (EEG), a tool that measures electrical activity in the brain, they had studied patients with delirium and concluded, "Not only does the presence of delirium often complicate and render more difficult the treatment of a serious illness, but also it carries the serious possibility of permanent irreversible brain damage." It seemed a prescient statement forty years ahead of its time and solidified my drive to investigate further. I couldn't get my concerns about delirium out of my mind—this connection between critical illness and possible brain injury. The lung was my organ of expertise, yet the mysteries of the brain called to me. For a pulmonologist to think about this was unconventional. When I wrote in my new research notebook, "Hypothesis: the lung bone is connected to the brain bone," it almost felt like a betrayal.

The seed of the idea was planted a couple of years earlier when I was invited to attend a geriatric education retreat by Dr. Hazzard and Dr. Haponik, my two mentors from Wake Forest. They had organized a conference in beautiful St. John in the US Virgin Islands. Their hope was to draw attention to geriatrics, and they had gathered together many of the leaders in the fields of aging and critical care to facilitate discussions in advancing treatment for the millions of older people barreling toward illnesses that would likely land them in the ICU.

I was not among the original invitees, but on the Wednesday before the weekend gathering, a physician had to drop out. I was called in as a last resort to fill the time slot. With only one published paper to my name, I knew my place on this roster was dubious at best. Petrified, I stayed up for the next seventy-two hours straight, reanalyzing my data from my one paper, trying to figure out a way to make it relevant to geriatric medicine. Twenty percent of my patients in the study were elderly (seventy-five or older), and while they seemed to tolerate being liberated from the ventilator well, they were dying at a greater rate once they were discharged from the ICU. I decided to focus on this.

The underlying assumption was that their deaths could be attributed to lung failure related to their time on the ventilator, so maybe a specific weaning protocol needed to be developed for elderly patients. The more I delved into the data, however, the more I saw that this was not the case. All my patients in the study, regardless of age, had followed the same weaning protocol and had all been successful in breathing spontaneously when given the chance, when their lungs were ready. The older patients had all come off the ventilator and been discharged from the ICU just as quickly as the younger patients.

In my head, I invoked the metaphor of a horse race, all the horses leaving the gate together. Those who finished the race did so at around the same time. Only beyond the finish, the discharge from the ICU, did the older patients start to falter. Some died, and some returned to the ICU and were intubated again, sometimes more than once, and then subsequently died. While lung failure was the primary reason that all the patients had originally been admitted to the ICU, the data showed that something other than their lungs was causing older ones to die at a greater rate. The question was, what? I took long swims in the azure waters of Caneel Bay trying to come up with an answer.

When I gave my talk, many in the audience, as I had feared, greeted my findings with skepticism. Not only did I tell the group of critical care doctors, primarily pulmonologists, that the lungs were not the chief suspect, but I went one step further. I wagered a guess, a hunch, that it was the brain. "What are we supposed to do with this?" they asked. "Our focus is the lung!"

• • •

In many ways, the talk I presented in 1998 in St. John was a turning point for me, although I was only just beginning to piece my ideas together. My patients' delirium stories, arising from their time spent on a ventilator, finally forced my attention beyond the lung. But I was growing as a doctor. I didn't shift my gaze from one organ to another, switching the lung for the brain. Instead, I kept both within my view, and more important, I began to understand the central role a patient and his loved ones play in the narrative of his illness.

With the hypothesis in my notebook proclaiming the direction of my new research, I was ready to throw myself into discovering the connections between brain dysfunction, lung failure, and critical illness. It felt disloyal, in a way. I had spent the previous ten years enamored of critical care medicine for its lifesaving potential, channeling deeper into its world and honing my skills to take medical technology and expertise as far as they could possibly go. Esteemed colleagues had embraced my work and welcomed me into the culture, but now I was finding myself at odds with them. My new research ideas weren't popular with other doctors or hospital administrators. More than once I was asked, "Wes, *what* are you doing?" And my answers brought a fresh wave of headshaking and negative predictions: "This research is a dead end." "It won't be funded by the National Institutes of Health." "It's going to stunt your career. Pay attention to lung physiology and the science of the thorax."

I remembered from my college Latin that the word *delirium* comes from the verb *delirare*, a term used in agriculture to indicate when a plow is going out of the furrow. Having worked on a farm all those years, I had accidentally committed this cardinal sin when planting. But now, even though I was purposely veering off track, I felt disoriented and lonely.

I was a little scared, too, by what harvest my research would yield. My critical care patients were telling me that they had delirium, and my intent was to discover the cause, the long-term impact, and how to mitigate its effects. My gut feeling was that the answer to the first question lay with the very technology that we used to save our patients' lives. That thought was overwhelming.

In June 2000, as I dedicated myself to this new research, I stepped down from my position at the Vanderbilt Transplant Center and left the field of organ transplantation. It had changed me for the better as a doctor, had taught me to slow down, reflect, appreciate the here and now, but I hoped my research might help more people in the long run. I could cast a wider net with full-scale clinical trials, something that just wasn't possible within the limited scope of lung transplantation. I also admitted to myself that I wished my patients could live longer than they did with their new organs. Of the couple of thousand people who received lung transplants each year, only about 60 percent would be alive five years later, largely because of the ravages of chronic rejection. Although I marveled at transplant as a science and a phenomenon, I had reservations about the ticking clock we planted in our patients' chests. But that was the nature of the lung.

Ready to study delirium, I pulled out my favorite medical school textbook on the brain, not my beloved Guyton this time, but Eric Kandel and James Schwartz's *Principles of Neural Science*. It always gave me a thrill to open my old books and feel again that sense of excitement, that readiness to find new knowledge that had propelled me as a young doctor. My eyes fell on the twenty-five-hundred-year-old quote from Hippocrates printed on the first page: "Men ought to know that from the brain, and from the brain only, arise our pleasures, joys, laughter, and jests, as well as our sorrows, pain, griefs, and tears. Through it, in particular, we think, see, hear, and distinguish the ugly from the beautiful, the bad from the good, the pleasant from the unpleasant. . . . It is the same thing which makes us mad or delirious, inspires us with dread and fear, whether by night or by day, brings sleeplessness, inopportune mistakes, aimless anxieties, absentmindedness, and acts that are contrary to habit."

I paused at the word *delirious*. It felt like a sign, a green light for my research. I plunged into the text and found a classic phrenology map of the brain from the 1800s, showing areas that this now-debunked pseudoscience claimed would expand and contract, depending on development or regression of character traits such as benevolence, spirituality, and hope, sitting adjacent to regions for combativeness, persistence, and tact. I wondered immediately what swaths of our current thinking about the brain in critically ill patients might prove to be untrue.

I moved to what I knew to be factual: the anatomy of neurons, myelin sheaths, nodes of Ranvier, the electrophysiology of conduction, and the chemistry of synapses. This is the latticework of the mind, precisely what I worried was being damaged in my patients on ventilators. The brain was different from the organs that captured most of my attention in the ICU—kidneys, heart, liver, and lungs. It was more than the sum of its parts, the locus of identity and meaning for a person. When the brain became injured, we saw it in a patient's actions, thoughts, behaviors, and words. It was extraordinary.

· · ·

Once I started my research on delirium in the ICU with Brenda Truman (now Brenda Pun), a young nurse practitioner, I saw again how our well-intentioned technology silenced our sickest patients. Without their voices, we didn't have a way to measure accurately the presence of delirium. We created a tool specifically for patients on ventilators, building on work by Dr. Sharon Inouye and her colleagues, adding screening questions that enabled intubated (and thus nonverbal) patients to answer with a nod of the head or a squeeze of a hand.

In our first delirium study, Brenda and I enrolled 111 patients. Twice each day we checked for delirium by determining if they could pay attention and follow simple commands using our new Confusion Assessment Method for the ICU (CAM-ICU). "How are you today, Mr. Rowe? Can you look at me and squeeze my hand?" Then Brenda or I continued, "Great! Now squeeze my hand every time I say the letter *A*. If I say a different letter, don't squeeze. Ready? . . . C-A-S-A-B-L-A-N-C-A [or "A-B-A-D-B-A-D-D-A-Y"]. . . . Nice job, Mr. Rowe!" We counted every time patients squeezed on the *A*'s and did not squeeze on the consonants. Then we compared the results to the forty-five-minute psychiatrist's reference standard evaluation and determined that eight out of ten correct meant they were able to pay attention and did not have "inattention" and therefore were not delirious. We also showed pictures of everyday objects and asked a few more yes-or-no questions. In just thirty-seven seconds on average with each patient, we were able to assess whether delirium and the risk of brain injury were present. The soft press of my patient's hand felt like a huge connection as I looked into his eyes. It was him saying, "I'm in here. I've been here all along." When the patient was unable to squeeze my hand or pushed at the wrong time, it was an eloquent communication, too. A cry for help. I knew that he needed a different kind of medical attention.

One patient, Jessica, a young woman with advanced liver disease, confined to her bed for over two weeks, was so weak that she couldn't squeeze my hand. Instead, I asked her to bat her eyelashes once for an *A* and twice for other letters, then tested her for inattention, using the letter string *A-B-R-A-C-A-D-A-B-R-A*. She looked up at me with trust, and each time I said a letter, she slowly and methodically draped her long eyelashes, once or twice, across her eyes. Her perfect score showed me she didn't have delirium, which was important, but that was eclipsed by the far bigger lesson Jessica taught me. I saw her through that test. Along with trust, I had seen fear in her eyes, the need to connect with another human, ask questions, and hear some answers. I stayed at her bedside long after the testing was done, asking her simple questions that she could answer with a downward sweep of her lashes. In the middle of the high-tech world of the ICU, it was basic. Two humans communicating. It felt right. The need to determine if she was suffering from delirium had yielded greater gains than I had considered possible. In my quest to heal the lungs, I had discovered the brain and, beyond that, a glimpse of my patient.

• • •

Years after I had started on my odyssey into delirium, I read Ann Patchett's perspicacious novel, *State of Wonder*, about scientists traveling into the Amazon along an unforged path of discovery. I underlined a quote and have shared it with physicians at dozens of international critical care congresses: "Never be so focused on what you are looking for that you overlook the thing you actually find." I love that sentence. It's the exact process by which I found my direction.

Our CAM-ICU method was published in the *Journal of the American Medical Association* (*JAMA*) in 2001. *JAMA* editor and brilliant physician-scientist Dr. Deborah Cook played a vital role in championing delirium work at the journal, seeing it as a matter of human importance in critical care, even though late-adopter peer reviewers discounted the topic. Now translated into over thirty-five languages, the CAM-ICU is used all over the world for monitoring delirium in ventilated and nonventilated ICU patients alongside another popular instrument, the Intensive Care Delirium Screening Checklist, developed by Dr. Yoanna Skrobik from McGill University. The CAM-ICU was the foundation on which I built my research.

• • •

Before the 2020 pandemic quarantine, I attended an eye-opening post-ICU support group at the CIBS Center that reminded me of the central role delirium still plays in the lives of critically ill patients both in the ICU and when they return home. We had a large group of attendees, all our regulars sitting around the long table—Tommy, Janet, Lovemore, Mike, Richard, Sarah Beth, Kurtiss, Kyle, and Marylou—and several newcomers as well. The huge flat-screen that takes up the entire far wall was packed with faces as other survivors joined us by Zoom from around the country and across the world. Jan, Glynda, Steve, Sheila, and Ron. A couple of new additions there, too. Word of the group had been spreading. The session was run by Dr. Mina Nordness, a surgeon interested in the long-term effects of critical illness, and Dr. Caroline Lassen-Greene, a neuropsychologist especially concerned with quality of life in patients and caregivers.

"Sometimes the dreams come back," said Sarah Beth quietly. "Just out of the blue." She paused, thinking. Several people were nodding. We'd been talking about burnout, the exhaustion of living with ongoing critical illness, and being defined by it.

"It's disquieting because you think they've gone away and your life is normal again, but then they return and remind you that it's not," continued Sarah Beth. "It's as if, no matter how far in the past your illness was, you just can't get away from it."

"You're right, it all came back to me again yesterday, in the middle of the day," Kyle blurted out. He grabbed his wife's hand. "Our daughter Harper was home having a pajama day with us, and there I was with the jaguar again. It was so real I could feel the terror." His eyes were wide, remembering. Standing six feet one, he was movie-star good-looking, a young Cary Grant with dark hair and a stocky build. He grew up in Muldrow, Oklahoma, where he threw hay bales into the barn, became a high school football star, then turned to fighting fires, even using his strength to rescue people from crushed cars. Then one day his pancreas exploded due to a prescription heart medication, and he landed in the ICU at death's door. He was only in his thirties.

Nordness interjected, "Kyle, some here might not know the details of your ICU stay. Can you start with some of your 'lived' delirium experiences, which I say because, to you, they're so real that they don't seem like hallucinations."

"Retelling and unpacking these experiences can be liberating and validating," added Lassen-Greene. "Kyle, if you start us off, others can build on that."

Kyle nodded. He seemed eager to share. "Well, everything was in vivid color. So I'm on the ventilator and I woke up, and my wife, Katie, was sitting next to me trying to tell me what's going on. I looked over my shoulder, just glanced up to the right, and my monitor was there. But behind it I saw a black jaguar perched up in the corner in the pounce position, moving its tail real slow. I remember getting upset. Katie thought it was about the monitor and being hooked up and said, 'It's okay, it's helping you breathe,' but I was thinking, 'There's an apex predator in the corner. Are we really going to pretend this cat isn't about to pounce and tear us all apart?'" He paused for a moment. "I was convinced that if I took my eyes off it, then this thing was going to kill us all. My hands were restrained, so I couldn't even defend myself. That went on for about a full day, and everyone thought I was looking at the monitor. And that was upsetting because I was thinking, 'I'm not the crazy here, you guys don't see this thing?'"

Kyle's experience with delirium in the ICU was one of the worst I had seen in a long while. In addition to the black jaguar, he believed he was a crew member on a research vessel heading to the Arctic Circle to study sperm whales, and another time he thought the nurses were witches. After we removed him from the ventilator, his delirium quickly deteriorated into catatonia. His muscle movements froze, and he couldn't raise his arms. This condition is known as catalepsy and mitgehen. When we lifted his hand up into the air slightly, it stayed perched there or even continued rising involuntarily until it looked as if he were pointing to the top of the Batman Building of the Nashville skyline outside his window. He could keep that pose for hours. By the next morning he became completely mute. He appeared to be awake, but for thirty-six hours he did not speak a word. Later he told us that during his mutism he was flying an airplane, and the ICU monitors were his instrument panel.

"How real did the jaguar look?" I asked.

"As real as if the beast walked into this room right now. And that's the weirdest thing, how clear those hallucinations still are, and everything else is real foggy."

Kyle's voice was shaking, and Katie put her hand on his shoulder.

They had weathered a lot together. I'd been happy to hear them say once that they had grown closer because of it. Delirium is not an easy thing to handle.

"It's the stuff of Stephen King novels," said Sarah Beth, nodding.

"I dreamed I was drowning," added Richard. "In a font. A baptismal font."

The delirium stories flooded in. There were so many of them. One survivor on the Zoom screen had dreamed he'd been jailed for five years and his wife had died. The experience was so real for him that it took two years after surviving and getting out of the ICU to realize that this wasn't true, even though his wife was right there with him day in, day out, clearly not dead. Another shared a story of hearing gun-shots outside his room and having his fingers cut off to keep him from telling others about the drugs being sold by the nurses. Yet another spoke about the extraordinary lucidity of her dreaming as she tried to prove to her relatives how well she was so she would be allowed to leave the hospital. I was struck by how much pain and suffering they all had endured. How they opened up to one another. And how much it seemed to help.

"I never had any of that, the hallucinations of jaguars, or drowning, but I couldn't pay attention. To anything! I just remember brain fog and searching for words even when what I wanted to say was not that com-plicated. Like I had rusty gears in my head struggling to work."

Everyone turned to look at Lovemore Gororo. One of the youngest in the group, he seemed to have been adopted by everyone. An honor student from Zimbabwe, he had come to the United States on an aca-demic scholarship to attend college and had recently graduated from Vanderbilt law school. He and his wife, Dani, a PhD student studying human geography, were newlyweds when Lovemore decided to slip out at dusk to buy ingredients to make her special Valentine's Day cupcakes. Returning to his car, he noticed a man and the barrel of a pistol staring him down from thirty yards away, then he heard a shot.

He ended up in the ICU for a long time. His inferior vena cava, the large vein that carries blood from the torso and lower body to the right side of the heart, was blown wide open, and his liver, intestines, and spinal cord were damaged, too.

As I looked at him, a handsome guy with a big smile, I knew the bullet was still lodged in his spine, and that beneath his gray sweatshirt his body was still scarred, yet he had no trace of anger in him. He'd had to learn to walk again and still struggled with PTSD.

"That confusion is a kind of delirium," I told him. "It's actually the most common."

In his case, the symptoms were clear and he was diagnosed early in his stay. I had seen in his medical chart that the nurses had noted that he was unable to follow commands during their delirium test. However, that doesn't always happen. Even though critical care teams now are aware of the warning signs and dangers of ICU delirium, and test—or should test—each patient every day, we're still not as good at spotting the purely quiet kind that Lovemore suffered.

We know so much more about delirium now, and its long-term impacts on critical care survivors, than when I first started my research twenty years ago. We are actively on the lookout for it in the ICU. A form of acute brain dysfunction, we know it must be given the same attention as other organ system failures. Acute delirium affects between 50 and 80 percent of critically ill patients, and 10 percent of these patients remain delirious at the time of their hospital discharge. We define it as a disturbance of consciousness, the inability to pay attention, and a change in mental status that develops rapidly over a short time. It manifests in many ways and is most obvious when a patient, after being awoken from sedation, is aggressive, agitated, pulling out IV lines, and possibly hallucinating. This is the hyperactive kind, which makes up only about 5 percent of all the delirium we see in the ICU. Much more often, patients are quiet, minding their own business, and seem fine, if a little muddled in their thinking. They have hypoactive delirium, or swing back and forth between the two, which is what I see 95 percent of the time.

• • •

It can be helpful to consider consciousness as having two main components: arousal and content. Put simply, arousal is how awake a person is, and content is how aware a person is of his surroundings. With delirium, many patients have normal arousal, meaning they may be wide-awake, combined with an abnormal content of consciousness. That is why your sick mother in the ICU might look you straight in the eyes, yet think she is on a boat somewhere in the dangerous waters of the Bermuda Triangle. Or why Kyle might have glanced over his shoulder at his monitor and seen a lurking jaguar.

The formal definition of delirium has less to do with hallucinations or delusions and more to do with inattention, yet for many patients it is the hallucinations and delusions that remain long after their ICU visits are over. In some cases, a patient with delirium may experience delusional thinking directly related to her critical care treatment. Some patients dream about drowning or suffocating, which makes sense if they are struggling to breathe on a ventilator. Patients with restraints on their arms often believe they are being imprisoned or held against their will in an underground space. Routine health-care procedures can bring on terrifying thoughts of torture and harm: patients believe they are being assaulted, raped, and abducted by nurses or doctors as catheters and feeding tubes are inserted, bed baths are given, and MRIs are taken. This can lead to narratives questioning the motives of a patient's family and friends. "How can they allow such terrible things to happen to me?" the patient may ask. "Are they in on it, too?"

Other patients suffer chilling visual and auditory hallucinations. Rosa Allen, my patient from years earlier, was certain a child was float-ing outside the window of her fourth-floor ICU room, even while she could not remember that she had given birth to a new baby. Once, I had a middle-aged patient with sepsis who believed an army of ants were swarming up his nose and into his ears. In all my years of treating patients with delirium, I have only heard of one positive delusional narrative. A woman believed her golden retriever was lying under her hospital bed throughout her entire ICU stay, and his supposed presence helped her enormously.

Over the past fifteen to twenty years, we have become much better at preventing delirium, detecting it when present, and mitigating its effects, but it is still a huge concern. Many of our group attendees struggle daily with the cognitive impairments left in its wake. The week before, a survivor told us she had made a peach pound cake from a brand-new recipe, only to discover she had added with the butter its waxed-paper packaging. She had laughed at herself as she told the story, but her voice cracked, too. Though a small matter, it had shaken her sense of self and opened the void again, reminding her, she said, that her brain was not the way it used to be. She was broken.

Lovemore's PTSD stemmed both from his trauma and the delirium he experienced. Sometimes he had vivid, violent nightmares, even during the day, but those were beginning to happen less frequently. More often, he said, "It's like my mind doesn't fit inside my brain anymore. I know this sounds bizarre, but my mind is slightly off, the way the color of a shirt just doesn't go with someone's outfit, or like the smell of milk that, while not rotten yet, is clearly turning spoiled." It was as if he just wasn't himself anymore.

And for Kyle, his continued sightings of the jaguar still haunted him. When it appeared again the day before, he'd had to leave the room, shaking, terrified, and almost breaking down in front of his young daughter. His strength, sharing with his fellow survivors in the face of that fear, was lionhearted.

As the group wound down and the attendees started to leave, I went to give Sarah Beth a hug. She wasn't her usual bouncy self. She smiled her fabulous smile and shrugged. "Just having a down day. But I'm taking my dog Freddy for a long walk later. And I have a new book to read."

Kyle and Katie were still sitting, talking together. Both Irish, they were married about eight years earlier on Saint Patrick's Day so that they could celebrate their shared heritage. When I asked Katie if she had felt timid in advocating for Kyle during the overwhelming days of his ICU stay, she fired back, "Not at all. I felt empowered."

One of the things we discovered over the years is the important role a patient's loved ones play in bringing the patient's brain out of its disordered, delirious state, from inattention to attention. Dr. Sharon Inouye, a leader in geriatric medicine and aging research, reduced delirium in older hospitalized (non-ICU) patients—a 33 percent relative risk reduction—through multiple strategies. Interventions included cognitively stimulating activities such as playing word games or talking about current events; orientation to remind patients of their surroundings; sleep protocols such as a back massage, relaxing music, or keeping noise down; attention to vision and hearing by giving patients their eyeglasses or their hearing aids. We have built on these findings and adapted them for the ICU. So many of these activities can be carried out—and advocated for—by family members. It was Katie who believed Kyle when he babbled about the jaguar. She grasped how real his tortuous, delirious wanderings were to him and spoke up on his behalf to the nurses, allowing the concerns he couldn't voice to be addressed by the medical team.

"It was the scariest thing that ever happened to me," Katie said. "I was losing him. He was in this faraway place in his brain. It was like I was physically separated from him. But that had a rebound effect of bringing us tighter together because I saw . . ." She paused. "You see everything about a human being when they're in the ICU. Everything. Physical, mental, spiritual. I saw him go into the depths of delirium and then come out of it. You see a stripped-down person, and he was kind all the time. That's who he really is." Her voice choked up a little. "So, yes, it really brings you together."

• • •

During the coronavirus pandemic, a lack of family at the bedside exacerbated the incidence and duration of delirium, contributing to the long-term ramifications of this terrible disease. In our COVID-ICU, Shelley Fugate arrived at 1:00 p.m. sharp, just as she'd promised Ray she would. This was the sort of stability he needed. She took a deep breath, knocked on the door to his room, and he glanced away from the window and in her direction. She could see him clearly through the glass pane, and they beamed at each other. I could only guess her thoughts when she saw her husband, her valiant high school crush, laid so low, so unlike himself, but she didn't let anything show. She knew her job was to stand tall for him. She had to be the light his dysfunctional brain could move toward, creeping out of the shadows of its disordered thinking toward her, a familiar presence, a reminder of whom he used to be. Her voice needed to reach along their phone lines and find the heart of him, orient him, and give him hope even when she found herself without it.

I watched her start the call to Ray and saw that he was listening. I knew it must be hard for her to speak with a loved one when his brain was not working, when he was not the person she once knew. Delirium is excruciating and relentless. Yet, I could already see that Ray was looking calmer, leaning toward where Shelley was standing outside his room. His heart rate and blood pressure were lower now that his anxiety had lessened. I walked down the hallway to give Shelley and Ray some privacy on their call. Even with our latest technology, the best medicine could still be the presence of family. It's especially crucial in helping the brain to clear.

Chapter 6

The View from the Other Side of the Bed— Illness Revisited

> *Turning together to face what our patients face ...*
> *allows us to not only bear witness, guide our patients and*
> *treat disease, but also to bring more compassion to each*
> *moment, a compassion that extends even to ourselves.*

—Rana Awdish, *In Shock*

BY THE MIDDLE OF 2000, my wife, Kim, and I had lived in Nashville for two years, and it was beginning to feel like home. She had finished her fellowship training and was now a full-time pathologist at Vanderbilt, spending her days between patients and the lab, examining tissue samples looking for the presence—or absence—of cancer and other diseases. I, too, was filled with a sense of purpose, juggling my days in the ICU with my work in the clinic as a physician and as an investigator, designing a new study on delirium. We had just bought our first home, not too far from the hospital, and moved in with our children and our black Lab, Rex. We planted a cheerful patch of black-eyed Susans and coneflowers, while pale pink sweet azaleas bordered our back lawn. It felt good to be building something together, to be putting down roots.

During the hot summer months, we often took our daughters to a local swimming pool, fitting around our work schedules some much-needed family time. The girls were at an age when they seemed to be in a constant flurry of movement, and their energy and excitement sustained us, keeping us in the here and now, beyond the hospital walls.

One Saturday, as Kim oversaw the twins at the shallow end of the pool, I sat near the high diving board where our six-year-old swam and played with her friends. I watched as she moved in and out of the water, up the ladder, along the board, and then leaped back into the pool, sleek as an otter. The motion was mesmerizing. I was happy that she delighted in something I had enjoyed throughout my own childhood and did still, squeezing in early-morning swims as often as I could. As I dipped my feet in the water, I sensed a flash of pink out of the corner of my eye and turned my head. A child was falling from the diving board. My child. Fifteen long feet toward the pavement below. I heard the thud as her head hit the concrete, blood spilling, and watched her body crumple in on itself then flop, unconscious, over the edge into the pool. I plunged in and scooped her out, laying her gently on the hot cement like a broken bird. Her body was limp, but then reared up, fighting me, flailing and seizing, and as I held her, my fingers slid inside a two-inch split in her skull, touching ragged edges of bone. A fracture. I knew this was how lives changed in an instant. A line in the sand marking before and after. I raged, banging my fists on the ground, screaming, "Why? Why did this happen?" As I lifted my eyes, I saw Kim standing frozen, tears streaming down her face.

The five-mile ambulance ride to the hospital seemed interminable. I gripped Kim's hand, but we did not speak. I couldn't. The EMT radioed ahead, "We've got a six-year-old girl en route to the ED with head trauma and seizures." I held my breath while my mind spun in an endless circle of desperation and guilt. How could I have let my child fall? I had seen countless tragic accidents in busy emergency departments. I should have known better. I watched as she moved in and out

96

of consciousness, willing her to be okay, the scream of sirens drowning my thoughts.

When we arrived at the hospital, so familiar to us, we hurried after the EMTs as they rushed the gurney into the packed waiting room. The neuro team was ready and swarmed upon us, racing us into a room, setting up oxygen, monitors, ordering tests. My mind buzzed. I saw this play out every day, but this time it was different. Kim and I stood back, silent, watching, letting the doctors and nurses do their jobs.

The waiting was endless. It was as if time had crystallized into this one moment of not knowing, and I was sentenced to dwell there, never moving forward. Yet I could move backward in time, reliving the details of the day: the girls' fizzing excitement as we set off for the pool, the baking sun, the bright flowers in their planters, the flash of pink, the fall. I heard the thud over and over. Each time, I recoiled with regret and pain. I thought about the many ways a brain could not survive such a trauma. The pages of Kandel and Schwartz's *Principles of Neural Science* sprang to mind, and I saw detailed illustrations of the frontal, parietal, temporal, and occipital lobes and their accompanying functions: problem solving, emotional regulation, speech, memory formation, color processing, and more. Elements that make up the basics of what it means to be human. Would it all be taken away?

I realized I was not in control of the outcome. This devastated me, then liberated me. Since my childhood, I had always mapped out my next steps. When things went wrong, I knew how to find a way through, but now reason failed me. I began to hope in a way I'd never done before. Not for a specific outcome. And not as a parent or a physician. I hoped instead as a child does, fiercely, that everything would work toward the good, even if I was blind as to how. I abandoned any desire to control and eschewed intellect for acceptance of whatever lay ahead.

Finally, we were allowed up to the neuro-ICU, four floors above my own ICU, and ushered into one of the rooms. It was so familiar to me with its cardiorespiratory monitoring instruments, but it now seemed alien and frightening. I entered as a parent, scared of what I might learn within its sterile walls. My daughter looked so tiny in the bed, helpless in an oversize blue hospital gown and hooked up to a heart monitor and multiple IV lines. She squinted up at Kim and me, trying to keep her eyes open.

"It's okay, sweetie," said Kim, her voice soft. "We're here now." She leaned over the bed while I hung back. I felt clumsy and out of place.

"We have the CT scan results," said the neurosurgeon.

The words hung in the air. I caught Kim's eye and knew she felt the same dread that lay heavy in my stomach. She nodded.

"The foramen magnum is fractured in two places," he said. "It was a bad fall."

I sucked in my breath. It was the absolute thickest part of the bone at the base of the skull, where the brain stem joins the spinal cord. I had never even considered that her fracture would extend all the way through the foramen, much less on two sides.

"But the brain scans are clean. We are hoping she'll be fine."

I couldn't believe it. No subdural or intracerebral hemorrhage. I thanked the surgeon, hugging Kim, tears rolling down our faces. I vowed to myself to do better as a father. As a husband. As a physician.

We stayed in the ICU for three nights, Kim and I taking turns sleeping fitfully in our daughter's narrow hospital bed. Those were long expanses of reflection for me, as I became attuned to the daily routines of the hospital from this new perspective. I saw the way my daughter huddled into herself in her bed, as if by being invisible she might pretend that she was somewhere else instead. She seemed far from us in time and space, rarely opening her eyes or speaking, other than for temperature checks and the constant hourly neurological examinations. She seemed to exist in an in-between space.

During the night, I told her stories about a boy and girl called Ethan and Ally, my voice spooling across the space between us. I'd been making up these tales for my daughters for years, seeing myself as Ethan advising and guiding them through the world. Now I imagined this thread of normalcy, something from before the fall, connecting us to each other and to the world outside this room.

Often I dozed off, awaking to the noise of the machines as they dinged throughout the night, noting the way they invaded my dreams—how the bright lights of the monitors pierced the semidarkness, and how often I awoke not knowing where I was. Every time I heard the footsteps of doctors or nurses, their voices in the room, I startled, expecting bad news, even though I knew the neuro checks were stable. I worried that the CT findings weren't sensitive enough to see the underlying damage. That she might develop a delayed cerebral hemorrhage, and that surely there was extensive contusion of her cerebral cortex and cerebellum. I knew there was at least a possibility she wouldn't make it out of the hospital alive. I felt trepidation and a heightened sense of vigilance, as if now that fate had opened the door to critical illness within my family, it could never again be completely closed.

I had thought I understood what my patients and their loved ones endured when they came into the ICU, but now I saw how far my knowledge had fallen short. I had responded to their needs with my medical learning and technical expertise because I thought they were there just to be fixed. I believed families needed me to keep their loved one alive. And they did. Just as I needed my daughter to be kept alive. But they hoped for so much more. They were scared and wanted to be held, not physically, but in the gaze of the doctor, to be seen and heard and supported. They needed me to know that this hospital stay had barreled into their lives like a tornado, turning a mundane Tuesday into the unfathomable. They were vulnerable and afraid. They came to me wanting to be pieced together again, body and soul.

From our earliest days of medical training, we doctors are taught to examine patients from the right side of the bed, and I had always done so. Now, sitting on the left side, the family's side, I saw that the view from here was completely different. The neurosurgeons provided meticulous care, yet I felt shortchanged. I wanted them to see that in this ICU room, under their care, our lives teetered in the balance. The entire trajectory could change based on an image they might show us, or a sentence they might utter. Or more strikingly, what they did not say. I wanted to tell them that my daughter dreamed of becoming a dancer, but I was unsure how, so I stayed silent. I realized that my patients must feel this way, too. They needed me to make myself available in ways I had not yet considered or offered. If I'd once been hypnotized by the spell of science and technology, I was now waking up.

I found myself thinking about *The Doctor*, a painting I loved by the British artist Luke Fildes, inspired in part by the death of his young son. It was made into a postage stamp in 1947 to herald the centennial of the American Medical Association, later used in their fight against President Harry Truman's proposal for a national health-care system, and, ironically, used again just a few years ago to celebrate the fiftieth anniversary of the UK's National Health Service. In his masterpiece, created in 1891, Fildes illuminates two figures by lamplight, a critically ill child in the center and, on the left, a physician, elbow on knee and hand on chin, gazing at his patient, who lies in a makeshift bed in a cramped cottage kitchen. In the background, the parents look on with anguish. Just a few years earlier, as a young physician starting out in ICU medicine, I had scoffed at the image, thinking it antiquated and out of touch. I pitied the doctor who couldn't save the child simply because he didn't have the tools, not even antibiotics, at his disposal. But now I realized that this was the kind of doctoring I yearned for: the intent gaze, the connection between the doctor and his patient as he entered the family's life. I valued the extraordinary humanity in the doctor's expression as he questioned perhaps, "What more can I do?" or "How can I help this child?"

Some posit this painting was created as a reaction to public suspicion of the growing move toward overreliance on science in doctoring.

Then, as now, patients wanted their physicians to retain their humanity and tend to the sick by spending time at the bedside. Luke Fildes's doctor, painted by a man who knew the sadness of losing a child, seemed to be the embodiment of this ideal.

I began to see my daughter's hospital room through a new set of eyes. I noticed it was designed strictly with the treatment of physical disease in mind, and not for patient comfort at all. The bland walls stared back at me, uninspiring and devoid of artwork. There was nothing soft or colorful or remotely homey, nothing to warm the soul or distract us. In some ways, the curative aspects of the room were illusory.

Our ICU had introduced an open family visitation policy a few years earlier in the mid-1990s, way ahead of many other major medical centers, and I truly valued its importance now both for patients and their loved ones. I could well imagine how afraid and disoriented a patient would feel if left alone. As a child, my daughter had little understanding of her health-care treatment, and I started to see her as representative of my intubated, ventilated patients. She needed an advocate because of her age, whereas my patients needed advocates because of an inability to communicate, forced upon them by their illness, by life-support technologies, and by me.

When my daughter finally left the neuro-ICU, we headed home, ready to close that chapter of our lives. The doctors had assured us that the skull fractures would heal on their own and that normal life could resume. But I wasn't sure it would be that simple. Critical illness leaves a mark, even in the best of outcomes. For me, life seemed more tenuous. The outside world had intruded into the safe bubble of my family life. I was shaken as a husband and a father, in ways that were both obvious and confusing. There are no discrete boundaries to the impact of life-threatening illness.

I devoted myself to more time at home with Kim and the girls, breathing in the small moments that bound us all together: watching Rex career through the backyard chasing rabbits, telling the girls at bedtime the adventures of Ethan and Ally, and sitting with Kim on the patio as days faded into soft nights. In time, I channeled myself back into my job as well, fired up to understand the way my patients' brains were damaged by delirium and what that meant for them when they left my care. I resolved to remember the view from the left side of the bed.

Chapter 7

Deciding My Path—Combining Research with Clinical Care

> *In examining disease, we gain wisdom about anatomy and physiology and biology. In examining the person with disease, we gain wisdom about life.*
>
> —Oliver Sacks, *Awakenings*

EVER SINCE MY CHILDHOOD I had liked to go swimming, whenever possible, to think through my ideas. I was thrilled to discover that the neurologist Oliver Sacks swam whenever he could and cited his time spent doing so as especially productive. Usually, my morning-workout pool was full of swimmers, even before dawn, with people starting the day submerged in their own worlds, but today it was empty. Just me slicing through the water. I had come to the pool to process my thoughts and consider the next steps in my research, but as my arms pulled, lap after lap, my head echoed with the words "Critical care is causing harm . . . critical care is causing harm . . . I am causing harm."

It was the spring of 2003, and I had received the final data on a study that shook me to the core. I had designed an investigation to understand the relationship between delirium, length of hospital stay, and death in ICU patients receiving mechanical ventilation. The results were unequivocal. Delirium in the ICU predicted a higher likelihood of dying within six months, even after considering preexisting diseases and other new organ problems. It also forecast a longer hospital stay, elevated costs, and an almost ten times higher risk of cognitive impairment at hospital discharge.

I had stared at the figures: 82 percent of the patients—my patients—had developed delirium while in the ICU under my care, and, of those, 34 percent had died within six months, a tripling of the risk of dying compared to those who did not develop delirium. It dawned on me that we were saving people's lives in the ICU only to have them die later from something we might have created ourselves. Just a couple of years earlier we hadn't considered delirium important enough to measure; we told one another it was normal, a side effect of being in the ICU, of pushing back against death. We brushed it off. Yet now the data showed incontrovertibly that delirium was devastating to our patients' health. Questions raced through my mind. Which parts of our care choices were contributing to delirium? What did our patients' cognitive impairment mean for them after discharge? What could we change about our treatment, and how? As a doctor, I had always tried to hold myself to the higher standard of beneficence, doing good, rather than benevolence or wishing good. As I pushed through the water that morning, I could see how far I had fallen short.

Later, when I was on rounds discussing the details of my patients' care, I started to see potential harm in everything we did—from the hourly neuro checks that we imposed on our patients with brain injury, and that my own daughter had undergone, to the endless testing and blood draws and dispensing medications throughout the day and night. Our objective as physicians was to protect our patients, to keep them from harm, but what if we were impairing healing by interrupting the injured body's much-needed sleep? At what point did our actions and medications tip the scale from benefit to harm?

In the clinic, when I saw patients after discharge for return visits on wound healing or lung health check-ins, I started to ask about their experience of critical care. One of my former ICU patients told me he had felt shackled like a prisoner throughout his stay. "But I was guilty of no crime other than coming to you to get well," he said. To our team, his wrist restraints meant safety, but to him they were smothering. Demeaning.

Another told me of the existential dread he had felt while on the ventilator, the overwhelming sense of loneliness and captivity. "Like being in solitary confinement," he whispered, barely able to say the words out loud. I felt a lick of fear. Growing up in Louisiana, my friends and I had frightened one another with stories of the infamous Angola, the largest maximum-security prison in the country, just a few hours south of where we lived in Shreveport. We were terrified of crossing the law and ending up in solitary. It was the absolute worst thing we could imagine. I shook my head, apologizing. We had isolated him physically and spiritually. What role had this played in bringing on delirium?

"You saved my life, Doc," said my patient with a shrug. "I'm not complaining, just sharing."

I began to schedule my ICU patients for follow-up appointments so I could learn more about their stay. For some, the horrifying experience was something they hoped they would never have to repeat. Others had little recollection of it at all, which was also disturbing to them. Yet almost all of them added some variation of "But, hey, I'm still here, aren't I?"

I noticed that a few of my patients missed their return visits and had to call later to reschedule, or they showed up on the wrong day or at the wrong time. "I forget everything these days," said one, when I squeezed her in for an appointment between other patients. Another couldn't remember that she was supposed to be taking medications. When I asked how their jobs were going, most of them were still at home. "I just don't feel ready to go back to work." I started to hear those words all the time. Others had been fired because they couldn't do their job anymore or had embarrassing encounters in meetings, forgetting long-term clients' names, or presenting data incorrectly. Was this what cognitive impairment looked like? I realized that my rosy vision of their lives beyond my care was far from the reality. I thought back on my transplant patients and how we had expected their recuperation to take time, and the ways in which we had supported them, even prepared them in advance for the difficulties of their recovery. But then, despite the complexity of their surgeries, they had made progress and reentered their lives. For my critical care patients, survivorship was a very different story. It seemed that they couldn't shake the vestiges of their hospital stay.

"I sometimes feel like I'm just a good outcome for doctors," said one. "I may still be alive, but I don't feel like I'm living anymore."

• • •

I had tried to block out the chatter, the barrage of questions from friends and colleagues asking what I wanted to be: a clinician or a researcher. They said I couldn't be both, and Vanderbilt's date to finalize a choice of one track or the other was looming. In reality, one was never a pure clinician or researcher, the split was around 80:20, but I was torn between the two. I had come to love my role at the bedside. I longed to be a committed doctor with my eyes on the patient, but I feared it might be too time-consuming and would draw me away from my family when they needed me most. Those who chose the clinician route ended up spending so many hours at the bedside that their time split was more like 100:20, which comes at a high cost.

The path toward being predominantly a researcher was tempting for many reasons. In some ways, I felt I could make the most impact there, investigating ideas that would help patients globally. The thought of addressing original hypotheses, uncovering new data, and publishing findings to calibrate the field of medicine was exhilarating to me. I also knew I would find it difficult to see the problems my patients faced and not have enough time for research to create meaningful change.

In speaking with my mother about my indecision, she did what she has so often done and directed me toward literature. At her urging, I dove into Sinclair Lewis's 1925 novel, *Arrowsmith*, immersing myself in the story of physician-scientist Martin Arrowsmith, feeling the sense of absolute purpose with which he followed his art, seeking truth through science at every turn. I saw nobility and transcendence in his dogged pursuit of research, in the faith that he would find answers that could change medicine for the better. If I had to choose between being 80 percent clinical or 80 percent research, and I knew I did, following in Dr. Arrowsmith's footsteps was alluring.

I had just taken on my first mentee, Dr. Pratik Pandharipande, who was in his early thirties and had joined our faculty in Nashville after medical school in Mumbai, India, by way of a residency at a small hospital in New Jersey. Dr. Jeff Balser, chair of the Department of Anesthesiology, had asked if I would mentor Dr. Pandharipande, and I was excited, honored by his trust. I felt ready to provide guidance and support to a fellow doctor's hopes and aspirations. I was also nervous about the amount of work it might entail. At our first meeting, Dr. Pandharipande had appeared eager and forthright. As we spoke, I noted how humble he was, and gracious, and that he possessed the most important traits of all for a scientist: curiosity and an awareness that he didn't know everything. As Richard Feynman, the brilliant physicist, once said, "If we want to solve a problem that we have never solved before, we must leave the door to the unknown ajar."

Dr. Pandharipande was resolved to learn everything I knew about doing clinical research in the ICU, and his single-mindedness was helpful to me as I was trying to finalize my own choice. He had little academic training and knew that he would have to pursue an advanced master's degree or a PhD to build a research toolbox. We would have to meet for countless hours of counseling and teaching sessions on top of his already busy schedule. As I told him this, he nodded vigorously, his eyes shining. He couldn't wait to get started.

• • •

I was still pondering my path when Sarah Beth Miller came back to see Dr. Jim Jackson and me for an MRI of her brain. I still remembered the look on her face when she saw how drastically her IQ score had dropped after her ICU stay, revealing to her—and us—how far her new normal was from her old self. It opened my eyes to the way an experience with delirium and the subsequent cognitive impairment can change a life. How what seems like a little forgetfulness and fuzzy thinking could lead to early retirement, depression, or both. Dr. Jackson and I planned to compare Sarah Beth's new imaging with the MRI taken at the beginning of her ICU stay a few years earlier to understand whether her brain anatomy had changed, and if there would be a visual manifestation of her ongoing cognitive impairment. If so, as with the IQ test, we would have another before-and-after result to chart the parameters of her decline.

We had been waiting a while for the new MRI because Sarah Beth had splurged on metal braces after her hospital stay, and it wasn't safe for her to go inside a magnetic tube. She'd said, "If I can no longer win a quiz bowl, at least I'm going to dazzle with my smile." Finally here she was, with the braces removed, cheerful as usual and eager for her test.

I soon had the results in hand, and what I saw was devastating. Her previous scan had not shown any signs of brain atrophy, loss of brain tissue, but this new imaging, according to the neuroradiologist, looked "like the MRI of a demented eighty-five-year-old." Sarah Beth was fifty-two.

As anyone who observes a drawing of a brain quickly notices, the outside has a wrinkled appearance made up of bumps and grooves. These are the gyri and sulci. And on the interior, spaces called ventricles are filled with cerebrospinal fluid. This fluid courses down from the inside of the brain into the spinal canal, and it's what doctors drain with a needle when we do a spinal tap to look for meningitis or a bleed. Since the skull encases all of this in a fixed amount of space, our heads are filled with varying amounts of brain tissue and fluid. As I stared at Sarah Beth's latest MRI, I saw immediately that she had lost a huge amount of actual tissue. The sulci were much deeper, and the ventricles filled with fluid were larger, having grown to fill the void left by disappearing brain tissue. Millions of brain cells were missing. It was as if tons of rich soil had been removed from a garden, leaving behind puddles of muddy water and a few wilted perennials. Two areas of her brain showed especially significant degeneration, the hippocampus and the frontal lobes, regions that specialize in memory and executive function. This made sense. She had told us about her forgetfulness and her inability to organize her life. It was sickening to look at, yet I couldn't pull my eyes away. I saw the scan of Sarah Beth's badly damaged brain as a map of her muddled and tangled thinking. Visible confirmation of an invisible illness.

With Sarah Beth's imaging in hand, I knew I had to find solutions to my questions about why our critically ill patients were experiencing so much delirium. I needed to get at the truth. Her scan was showing me more than a picture of mild cognitive impairment: it was more severe. Was the neuroradiologist's assessment right? Was she now demented? Could that be possible? I shook my head as if to send the thought flying, but it was in my mind now and unlikely to leave until I addressed it. I also knew that I had made a decision. I would follow the research track. Already I was thinking about a neuroimaging study that would take MRI images of critical care patients so that we could know if their brains, too, looked like Sarah Beth's. But there was still the crucial question: What was causing delirium?

• • •

I developed two rules for myself as a physician-scientist to determine whether a question asked in the hope of improving medical care was worth pursuing. The first was, either answer must matter. I once had a mentee who wanted to study transfusing blood into ICU patients with delirium to see if improved oxygen transport to the brain would help clear their thinking. I didn't think it would work, but that is not why I advised against it. Since no one was doing this in practice anyway, a negative study wouldn't change medicine. So only a positive result would matter, breaking my first rule for research. My second rule was, study what you have a lot of. It didn't matter if an idea would be beneficial to patients unless we could find enough patients who met the study's enrollment criteria. Only when both rules were met did I chase an idea. This was very much the case with delirium. Very little research existed in this area, so I was confident that whatever we discovered would be valuable. I also knew that we would have no trouble finding enough patients to fill our trials. We had oceans of delirium in ICUs all over the world.

Unfortunately, my strides in this direction were met with resistance. My grant applications and papers were resoundingly rebuffed by multiple journals and funding agencies such as the NIH and Department of Veterans Affairs Merit Awards.

"This focus on delirium doesn't belong in the field of critical care," said leading neurologists and other reviewers at numerous highly respected journals, responding like a tragic Greek chorus. In variations on a theme, many professors told me there was no hope for academic success, funding, or making a difference with further research into delirium. Even though I was counseled not to take this personally, I did. Could they really think critical care doctors had found out everything we needed to know about delirium? Or did they still refuse to see the connection between the ICU, delirium, and brain injury? I started to dread opening my mailbox. Once again, I remembered all the people who had told me not to go down this research path. Maybe they had been right after all.

I felt unsettled. I'd had this same feeling in the past when I wasn't sure which direction to take, but this was different. Now I had made a choice. I had committed to the research track, and found myself thwarted. I wondered how many other researchers failed to get funding for their projects, and what happened to them. I was sure I was failing myself, my family, and my patients. Without funding for trials or publication of papers in high-impact, peer-reviewed journals, I knew it would be almost impossible to change medicine for the better.

• • •

During this time of uncertainty, I received a letter from Diane Whitten-Vile. Her sister, Donna Hilley, had spent ten days on the ventilator in our ICU, wrestling with septic shock. I remembered that she had struggled terribly with delirium, not knowing where she was or recognizing the visitors to her room. She was a CEO on Music Row in Nashville who oversaw multimillion-dollar music-catalog purchases and organized dinners for Washington's elite. We had played country music for her in her ICU room—John Prine, Bonnie Raitt, Marty Stuart, and Merle Haggard—trying to reach inside her mind and bring her back to herself while she lay sedated. I had felt good about the healing nature of music and started suggesting it to nurses caring for other delirious patients. I had always loved John Prine's music, particularly his songwriting, which seemed especially apropos: "Old people just grow lonesome / Waiting for someone to say, 'Hello in there, hello.'" Although I did ponder what Donna might make of some of the lyrics: "You're up one day and the next you're down. / It's half an inch of water and you think you're gonna drown."

Donna survived and was discharged. But now her sister wrote, "After she developed delirium, we couldn't seem to get her mental clouding cleared for months. She has tried to go back to work, although she cannot seem to fully bounce back. I saw her about a month ago, when she came to my daughter's Bat Mitzvah. She's lost her 'spark.' She was such a personality pre-illness, so gregarious and really the life of the party, but she is very flat now. She has memory problems, some long-term, but mostly short-term. She doesn't remember anything about her illness or her hospitalization. She looks much older, like an elderly woman now, and walks very slowly, always holding onto railings. She is fragile and vacant. The illness really changed her."

I sat at my desk with this letter for a long time. Donna Hilley was one of the patients enrolled in my study who proved that delirium was tightly linked to subsequent death and long-term cognitive impairment. Her spiral down into delirium was recorded in my files, a piece of data that, when aggregated with other data provided by patients like her, had helped us show the negative effects of delirium. That was important. But what did the data mean—numbers on a page and words in a journal read by people in health care—to the lived experience of my patients? Well, this letter told me.

Delirium changed people's brains and altered their lives. They came into the ICU one way and left heading along a completely different trajectory. One day they were living full lives, and the next they were clinging to a railing, barely holding on to their memories. I imagined that an MRI would have shown Donna's brain to have the same atrophy as Sarah Beth's or worse. I thought of Donna and Sarah Beth, and I remembered Teresa Martin all those years before, the young woman who had returned to my care in a wheelchair. Her befuddled thinking and limited life after her ICU stay made sense to me now. I was sure that if I found Teresa's medical file, the notes would include ICU psychosis and no mention whatsoever of delirium.

It saddened me that I hadn't truly seen the way Donna struggled after leaving our ICU. We had followed up with patients in the study six months after discharge and asked them a battery of neuropsychological questions and noted their answers, and at the time I thought that was a great improvement over what we used to do. But it wasn't enough. I remembered that Donna had seemed frail and looked older than her age. Had I known she was "larger-than-life" before her stay? Did I realize she had foundered in her job? It seemed that we were still missing a lot. Surely I could have helped her in ways after discharge, and the others whose lives must have been affected, too. I thought back on the numbers in my study, the 82 percent of patients who had developed delirium. What did their day-to-day lives look like when they made it back home? Were they able to return to their jobs or drive or socialize? These thoughts both sickened and galvanized me.

In that moment, I understood that while I had chosen the research track, my lab would be the ICU. I would have to study every aspect of what happened to my patients as their experience in the ICU helped me develop my research questions. Yet I was a clinician, too. I needed to be at my patients' bedsides during their ICU stays to tend to them in the present, and to support patients like them in the future. And I wanted to find a way to be there for them after discharge. From the start, I had committed to help those without a voice. Now more than ever, I needed to make my own voice heard and tell people about delirium. It mattered.

Chapter 8

Unshackling the Brain—Finding Consciousness in the ICU

I came awake on the fifth day. My first memory is that of floating up from the ocean bottom, my eyes still water-logged with what felt like scuba gear stuffed in my mouth and throat. I couldn't speak. As I broke to the surface, I understood that I was still in the ICU at Our Lady, but I heard nothing of what anybody said.

—Abraham Verghese, *Cutting for Stone*

IT WAS A COLD and rainy week in Nashville, and night seemed to close in earlier each day. I was taking care of Mrs. Noy, an older woman who had arrived in the ICU already on a ventilator. Her lungs were severely scarred with advanced idiopathic pulmonary fibrosis, and her chest X-ray reflected this, looking as if a blizzard had stormed in and settled there. Her prognosis wasn't good. Despite the team's best efforts she still wasn't responding to our barrage of steroids and antibiotics. With this disease, once a patient was on a ventilator and not improving, death was almost a given. I had invited her husband, a slight and silent man, on rounds with us every day, and he had watched us care for his wife. Now he sat by her bed holding her hand, looking apprehensive. I nodded at him and scooted in beside him, saying a few words. I knew Mr. Noy didn't always understand everything I said. He and his wife were originally from Laos, and while apparently she was fluent in English, he was not. This limited our conversations, but I did the best I could, explaining what we were doing to try to help his wife. I had asked for a translator on multiple occasions but was told the hospital didn't have anyone who spoke the Lao language, so I turned my attention back to my patient's medical care. As I sat by her bedside, the rain lashing against the windows of her room, she seemed so far away, deep down in another world.

The next day, her condition was worse, and I had to turn up her oxygen. As I looked at the images of her ravaged lungs, I shook my head. It wasn't what I had wanted to see. I showed Mr. Noy the images, comparing them to the earlier ones, and the difference was starkly visible. They confirmed what the rest of her labs and vital signs were telling me: the disease had overwhelmed her body. It was time to consider removing life support and shifting toward comfort measures. I needed to convey this to Mr. Noy, but I wasn't sure how. With the language barrier, it would be challenging to navigate such a nuanced and difficult conversation, yet without such a conversation, his wife's dying process might not be what she would have wished. Mr. Noy and I both needed more information. I had just read a paper on ethics consultations in the ICU, especially around end-of-life issues, and could see how useful the extra help and guidance would be in improving communication and avoiding conflict. I called the hospital's bioethics consultant. Immediately, she scoured Nashville and the surrounding areas and tracked down a translator who sat with Mr. Noy and eased him into the reality that his wife was actively dying.

Finally, after being provided low-dose morphine and being removed from the ventilator, she died a peaceful death with Mr. Noy at her side, stroking her hand and whispering into her ear. I thought we had reached the best overall resolution of a complicated situation. But when I doubled back with the bioethicist, I learned about the compounded anguish Mr. Noy had suffered during her illness. He had felt excluded, not knowing the details, not being able to process them, to understand what his wife was going through. I had tried to make it work, but without a translator, it wasn't good enough. That seemed so obvious now. I would learn that this unfairness around knowledge is referred to as epistemic injustice. How could I have thought that being included on rounds to watch doctors and nurses treat his wife, or being shown medical imaging, meant that he understood what was going on? Did I think that our knowledge as experts somehow made up for his lack of knowledge? The medical team possessed a vast universe of facts and data about his wife's illness and upcoming death, and intentionally or not, we had kept them to ourselves.

We had silenced our patient through our treatment and discounted her husband's role. Only when we reached the end had we asked ourselves what information he might have for us that could help his wife. We had allowed limited knowledge to flow from us to him, and even less from him to us. Whenever I think back on Mrs. Noy, my mind combines the rainy Nashville weather and the snowstorm in her lungs, and I see her at a great remove, silent, still, and underwater. With her husband drowning in incomprehension, voiceless and scared.

In many ways, this was the image I held in my head of most of my critically ill patients. Not when they were through the worst of their illness and off the ventilator, and able to sit up in bed and talk to me, but before that. When they were unconscious. They seemed so helpless. I thought of the quote "The true measure of a society can be found in the way it treats its most vulnerable members," attributed to many over the years. I needed to find a way to reach not only my vulnerable patients but those in other ICUs around the world. The scientist in me knew the most successful path must be through proving the best way forward.

• • •

By 2005, my team was midway through two randomized controlled trials: the ABC (Awakening and Breathing Controlled) trial and the MENDS (Maximizing Efficacy of Targeted Sedation and Reducing Neurological Dysfunction) trial. Both of these studies looked into ways to change highly ingrained, standard-practice patterns in the ICU. I had surmised that sedation might be causing problems for our patients and was investigating this hypothesis in two different ways.

In the ABC trial, with patients enrolled in Nashville, Philadelphia, and Chicago, we were reducing overall exposure to the standard drugs—benzodiazepines and propofol—so that patients would not be as deeply unconscious for as long. The patients were randomized, like the flipping of a coin, so that half of them had the drugs turned off every day and were allowed to wake up. If nurses assessed that the patient still needed sedatives, the patient would be restarted at half the previous dose, as the protocol dictated. Next, respiratory therapists turned off the ventilator every day so that patients could breathe unassisted. This two-step intervention was built on my first study, in which we turned off the ventilator daily, and that of Drs. J. P. Kress and Jesse Hall, who had pioneered shutting off sedation once a day.

In the MENDS trial, half our patients were receiving conventional ICU drugs, while the others were being sedated with a different drug completely. In many ways this was the riskier trial because since the 1980s everyone in critical care had always used benzodiazepines for sedating ventilated patients. There was rarely a question of using anything else. First developed in the 1950s, benzodiazepines, or benzos for short, became commercially available in the 1960s, and by 1977 they were the most prescribed drugs in the world. Diazepam (Valium) is probably the best known, but we chose to work with lorazepam and midazolam. We used them almost without thinking.

I had started to ask myself why we never questioned our standard practice of sedation. Why had I never speculated what it might be like for the body, the brain, to have a continuous flow of such powerful drugs coursing through them for days, even weeks, on end? A former ICU patient had come to see me in the clinic for follow-up of her emphysema, and I had ordered a breathing test and chest X-ray, and adjusted her inhalers. I asked my usual questions about her memory, how she was adjusting to her new post-ICU life, and was pleased to hear that she was doing much better, driving again, and had just dropped off her grandson at nursery school, something she hadn't done in months. "But," she said, "I'm having nightmares. Can you help me with that? I'm dreaming about drowning." She paused. "On the ventilator, I thought I was drowning. That you'd put me underwater and were drowning me. I know it sounds silly but . . ." She shrugged, struggling.

It didn't sound silly. I'd had similar thoughts myself, not about drowning, but about my patients going underwater as I sedated them, watching them drift down, down into unconsciousness. Until they were so far down I couldn't see them anymore.

My patient's story stayed with me over the next weeks, and as I sedated each new patient, I spoke to them in a reassuring way, telling them exactly what was happening to them, hoping to alleviate their fear. I wasn't sure if it would help. And I still couldn't shake the image of them being submerged. Tugged down as if they had a huge weight chained to their ankles, right when they were most vulnerable.

I had just finished reading Saul Bellow's novel *Ravelstein,* a wonderfully meandering story of friendship, old age, and the imminence of death. One paragraph especially stood out for me: "I was now the dying man. My lungs had failed. A machine did my breathing for me. Unconscious, I had no more idea of death than the dead have. But my head (I assume it was my head) was full of visions, delusions, and hallucinations. These were not dreams or nightmares. Nightmares have an escape hatch. . . ."

I hooked my patients up to a drip and sent them into the depths of unconsciousness, into a world of endless delirium dreams, and only let them surface when I thought they might be better. When their bodies might be healed. But in the meantime, and sometimes it was weeks, where were they exactly, and what was happening to their brains?

I knew well that being intubated and started on a breathing machine was painful and frightening for my patients, especially in the throes of all the other terrors of critical illness, and that painkillers and sedation were crucial to the patients' initial stabilization on life support. But I questioned the next few days of care. How long did patients need to be sedated, and how deeply unconscious did they have to be? At the beginning of the twenty-first century we didn't know the answers to these questions, despite our extraordinary advances in medical technology, and had little clue about our patients' depth of sedation.

• • •

The first surgical operation performed under a general anesthetic is widely accepted to have taken place on October 16, 1846, at Massachusetts General Hospital. A local dentist delivered ether vapors to twenty-year-old Edward Gilbert Abbott using a specially created tool and instructing him to inhale deeply. Within minutes, the young man was unconscious, and the surgeon was able to operate and stop the blood flow to a benign tumor. On awakening after his surgery in what is now known as the Ether Dome, Abbott is said to have remarked, "Feels as if my neck's been scratched." The procedure had been pain-free, an astonishing achievement in surgery, which had previously relied on alcohol, opium, and tying the patient down to get through operations.

From this auspicious beginning, the discipline of anesthesia moved forward, enabling more and more complicated—and time-consuming—surgeries and medical procedures to take place without pain. At the outset, doctors had to be careful not to kill their patients by overdosing them. Over time, as new drugs and new delivery methods were introduced, this became less of a concern. Doctors started to err on the side of administering more medication than necessary to ensure their patients were completely unconscious.

In 1963, Dr. Edmond "Ted" Eger developed a clinical tool called the minimum alveolar concentration (MAC) to gauge the level of anesthetic gas in patients' lungs. While it was widely adopted in the operating room for the management of millions of patients every year, in critical care we still tended to focus on our patients' physical signs to assess their level of unconsciousness, rudimentary as that seemed. Many ICUs still used the Ramsay scale, which was not ideal because it wasn't nuanced enough to assess complex patients and often provided conflicting readings from nurse to nurse. Others were using Dr. Curt Sessler's Richmond Agitation-Sedation Scale (RASS) or Drs. Richard Riker and Gil Fraser's Sedation Agitation Scale (SAS). I called Dr. Sessler, and together we designed and completed a large study to revalidate and integrate the RASS. It measured a patient's precise levels of arousal and sedation with Level 0 being "alert and calm," Level +4 as "combative," and Level –5 as "unarousable," one step lower than Level –4, which was "deep sedation." My concern lay with these lower levels. While we could accurately distinguish a stepwise descent of our patients into unconsciousness, once they were no longer responsive to voice or a painful physical stimulus such as a sternal rub, we lost track of their brain altogether. We knew they were unconscious, but had no idea exactly how far into the caverns they had descended. It brought me back to my water metaphors. Were they five feet under or ten or fifty? It was impossible to be precise. Or to know what was safe. Our trials were hoping to answer some of these questions.

• • •

One summer day, about two years into the ABC trial, I headed across town to check in on things in the ICU at Saint Thomas, a private hospital in Nashville. They were part of our study, as their research foundation had funded us—I was still receiving the all-too-familiar rejections from the NIH and the VA for my grant applications. I loved going over to Saint Thomas. Their four ICUs were always bustling, more open and louder than ours at Vanderbilt. I was an observer there, taking in the urgency, the split-seconds-matter atmosphere, while not being immersed in it. That day I ran into Jan Dunn, our main research nurse. In her late forties, with a friendly countenance and a soft voice, she was a staple there. We had hired her because she knew everyone and people believed in her. We had suspected that the trial, with its hands-on attention to turning off sedation and ventilators, and coordinating nurses and respiratory therapists to work together, would prove an uphill battle. In many ways, we had been right. I had come to know Jan well and appreciated her hard work, especially the way she rallied the teams and families.

Today she sighed and shook her head. "You know it's not working, right?" She pointed to her patient. He was profoundly sedated. "He's in the intervention group. But look at him. He should be awake by now."

My heart skipped a beat. He looked as if he were fifty feet down. I glanced back at Jan. "What do you mean?"

"Well, when the protocol directs nurses to turn the sedatives off, they do it for a little while, and then too often they turn them right back up. Like with this patient."

A wave of distress washed through me. But then, as I turned to look around the ICU, I saw several of the ventilated patients uncharacteristically awake. An elderly man peered up at the TV, while a woman across from him was listening to a young man in a Titans cap, maybe her son. I poked my head inside the adjacent patient's room and saw a woman propped up on pillows, reading, while the ventilator pushed air into her lungs. She gave me a tiny wave of her hand. I glanced back at Jan. Perhaps she was overly focused on her one patient who was still sedated rather than seeing the other patients who weren't. It certainly felt to me as if something different was happening here.

Sometimes I was frustrated that research studies and trials took so long to monitor and come to fruition, as I wanted change to happen more quickly for patients. I was seeing more and more people coming back to us after discharge from the ICU, glad to be out of the hospital but bewildered that they didn't have the energy to walk their dog, couldn't do the simplest crossword puzzle, or jumped with fear at the beep of a microwave. They were finding me through our website, medical conferences, and word of mouth. It seemed random, yet was steadily growing. While our team's work was focused on trying to prevent or lessen these outcomes, I could see that patients also needed support and interventions beyond their ICU stay. It seemed like a never-ending cycle.

• • •

I was hoping that the MENDS study would show that sedating patients more lightly would be better for them both in and out of the ICU. We were using a new drug, one that I had never heard of until I stumbled upon it a couple of years earlier while traveling to Dallas for a meeting with a pharmaceutical company, a last-minute replacement for my boss, Dr. Gordon Bernard. I had joined the usual gathering of executives, product managers, and representatives in an oak-paneled hotel boardroom. They were presenting their new sedative, dexmedetomidine, and I watched videos of patients receiving the drug. One was in the ICU, and she looked just like my patients, eyes closed and completely unconscious. I began to wonder if I might make the earlier flight home. But then the video showed this same ICU patient waking up when a doctor said her name, looking at him, listening, and following commands before falling unconscious again when he left her side. She was easily arousable, even while actively receiving the drug. This was totally unheard of and completely unlike benzodiazepines. Under their effect, patients would not emerge from sedation while receiving the medication. Even when the drip was turned off, they could take several hours or more to drift into consciousness. I started considering if this new drug might work for lighter sedation in a trial and urged the executives to consider this potential. I spoke to them with passion about ICU delirium and cognitive impairment, but I couldn't get through to them. They said their drug wouldn't make patients deeply sedated the way ICU doctors wanted. That was exactly my hope. I couldn't blame them for not seeing my vision. Benzodiazepines, and to a lesser extent the shorter-acting sedative propofol, had a viselike grip on the critical care world.

As I left the meeting, slightly demoralized and heading for the airport, a woman strode toward me and introduced herself as Yvonne Harter. She had just assumed global responsibility for dexmedetomidine, and so far, the company had not sold a single vial. The drug's coinventor and main thought leader, Dr. Mervyn Maze, was not answering her phone calls, and she seemed to be in as much need of inspiration as me. Yvonne told me she was curious about what I had said and asked if she could visit Vanderbilt. It felt like the beginning of something.

A few weeks later, I was happy to show Yvonne around Vanderbilt's medical and surgical ICUs. With permission from each family, I took her to see patients lying in dense comas and contrasted them with those who were awake. I could tell she saw how meaningful that difference was. "It's as if he's not in the room with us," she said about a patient in a drug-induced coma. "My mom's a nurse. She didn't finish high school, but after I was grown, she went back and got her GED and a nursing degree."

I walked Yvonne through the steps of the CAM-ICU, showing her that while our patient Mrs. Markson seemed quiet and obedient, she was delirious, and I explained why this was dangerous. "Delirium is like a canary in a coal mine, alerting me to damage going on inside her brain." I emphasized how the delirium piece of my patients' clinical courses could predict problems down the line in their lives, beyond the ICU, in countless negative ways.

She paused. "So, Dr. Ely, what I'm taking away is that here is an opportunity to help patients that wasn't on our radar. Let's see how to make it a reality."

As I worked with Yvonne, I learned that she had stared down risks and taken chances from an early age. She was born to parents from different cultural backgrounds, and when they divorced, her mom took her as a young child to poverty-stricken Oak Hill, West Virginia. They lived on food stamps and an abundance of mutual love and support for each other. "I never looked at my life as a hindrance," she told me. "Math and science provided endless adventures, and I went on to study chemistry and get the first college degree in my immediate family. From there, I just had to parlay my drive into a job where I could help other people." In her early twenties, Yvonne drove over a hundred miles to a pharmaceutical job fair and was stunned to find 350 people vying for 5 positions. A few days later she was one of the last ones standing, and the next day she began the career she loved.

As she walked out the swinging doors of our ICU, she turned and grinned. "Maybe you can get Dr. Maze to answer your calls."

It turned out that I could and we had even persuaded him to come to Vanderbilt. He had never thought about using dexmedetomidine to study something as nontraditional as delirium and the idea had excited him. Side by side, in a room overlooking the Nashville skyline, we had designed MENDS, a double-blind, randomized controlled trial, hoping to add one more puzzle piece to our plan to heal the delirium-impacted brain. Now, two years on, we would soon know the results.

• • •

Amid the rush and noise of the ICU, the sedated patients, silent and still, often seemed like an anomaly to me. In some ways, they were the calm at the center of the storm as well as the storm itself, while critical illness raged within them. During our MENDS study, I found myself gazing

125

at their placid faces, pondering what was going on in their brains and where they were exactly. As scientists, we still didn't have a real understanding of what happened at a physiological level when someone went from conscious to unconscious. As part of our study, however, our team was working with sleep experts to understand the exact depth of sedation for each of our patients. Or, as I thought of it, how far underwater they were. With a bispectral index (BIS), a computer-based, real-time monitor of brain function that had recently started to be used during surgery, we measured the electrical activity in each patient's brain via wires placed on her forehead. This generated an electroencephalogram (EEG)—essentially a detailed picture of the brain waves—which the BIS then translated into a discrete value ranging from 0 to 100, with 97 or 98 being the average for wakefulness, and between 60 (deep sedation) and 40 (coma) seen as the ideal sedation depth for general anesthesia.

We discovered something astonishing. The BIS scores on many of the patients sedated with benzos were well below 40, and some sank all the way down to 0, which was far beyond the threshold for coma. The corresponding raw EEG data, with their rippling horizontal lines that represented brain activity, told this same story: rapid scribbles for when the patient was awake, turning into less and less brain activity as they lost consciousness, moving beyond the point of being arousable, until there was just one long line of minimal electrical activity: a burst suppression. Flat line. Like a heart with no pulse. In my mind, it ran along the deepest ocean floor. Now I knew where my patients were when they were unconscious, and it was near death. We proved that burst suppression was a predictor of higher death rates. We were adding nails to a casket constructed from iatrogenic injury, harm caused by the medical treatment itself.

A couple of years earlier, a study by Dr. Deborah Cook in the *New England Journal of Medicine* had grabbed my attention. With her team, Cook had studied 851 patients in Canada who were critically ill on a ventilator and figured out what factors would lead doctors to withdraw life support and let someone die. The findings had shocked me: doctors were 3.5 times more likely to remove life support if they thought a patient had only a one-in-ten chance of ICU survival; 2.5 times more likely if they thought she might end up with severe cognitive impairment; and 4.2 times more likely if it was their "perception" that the patient would not want more life support. I knew that a heavily sedated ICU patient deep in a coma looked dead, and that this absolutely had to play a part in a doctor's thoughts. A wide-awake patient with sepsis looked much more alive and well—and therefore likely to survive—than a sedated and comatose patient with sepsis.

Dr. Cook's data showed that only 1 out of 10 of the 851 patients had a Do Not Resuscitate (DNR) order on admission to the ICU. Interestingly, by the time of death, 9 out of 10 patients had been designated DNR. It made me reflect on what role deep sedation may have played in those decisions.

Now I knew just how treacherously sedated our patients were, and how little brain activity they had. When I first read Dr. Cook's article, I thought about how many patients I may have inadvertently committed to an early death due to my use, or overuse, of sedation. Our BIS EEG data made me question again. I expressed my urgent concern to colleagues, but their response was "What are you talking about? Dr. Cook's article isn't about sedation." It was true that the word *sedation* didn't appear a single time in her paper. My colleagues were right in that sense, but I felt they were missing the big picture. We all were. I was sure that we needed to pay more attention to sedation.

• • •

Finally, in 2007, when the ABC trial was over and the data were analyzed, I learned that our intervention patients had received half the exposure to benzodiazepines as the usual-care patients—a stunning reduction. A huge experiment had indeed been conducted. Most of the time, stopping the sedatives had been easy and uneventful for the patients. We were thrilled to find that the experimental patients were liberated from the ventilator and discharged from both the ICU and the hospital four days sooner than the control patients (on a Monday, for example, instead of the following Friday). I thought of all the harm that could happen to an ICU patient in that time—new pneumonia, line infections, falls, pressure ulcers, blood clots—that was being avoided, yet I was still surprised when we calculated that 58 percent of those treated with our new wake-up-and-breathe ABC approach were alive at the end of one year, compared to only 44 percent of the patients treated with usual care, meaning a 14 percent increase in one-year survival. Billions of dollars could be saved with these shorter hospital stays, but I was most elated because for every seven people in the study, one more person was alive after a year. This was the first solid proof that reducing sedation in critical care could save lives.

We were excited to present our data on the international stage, but the next big meeting, the European Society of Intensive Care Medicine congress in Berlin, was scheduled in October when I would be in the ICU caring for patients. Instead of changing my plans, I asked my mentee, Pratik, to go. His father was so excited to witness his son's academic debut that he planned to fly from Mumbai to be there in person.

On the day of the presentation, Pratik called me immediately following his talk. His voice came over the line, stilted and wary. "I don't even know how to tell you," he mumbled, "but it didn't go well at all."

The audience had eaten Pratik alive. The French, Belgians, and Dutch had all said it was unethical to subject the control patients to days when their sedation wasn't shut off. They felt that equipoise—uncertainty within the medical community about whether a treatment will be beneficial—no longer existed. But we knew it did.

"The science already proved that turning off sedation gets them off the ventilator earlier!" they said. "We already turn off these medicines every morning," they chided Pratik, which was not true.

Pratik, though, so junior and deferential to these leaders in the field, had not mounted any defense for our trial. I imagined how differently things might have gone had I been there to argue against their claims. I would have reminded them that a just-published study of forty-four ICUs across France found that 95 percent of patients were deeply sedated on midazolam or propofol on days two, four, and still on day six of their ICU stays. The medical literature also had recent data from Canada, Germany, Brazil, the UK, and the United States documenting that not even a third of ICU patients in these countries were getting their sedatives turned off once a day. I felt terrible about the unanticipated reaction to our ABC study, and about Pratik's experience.

However, despite our group's weak showing in Berlin, the year ended well. After many evenings of talking science with Mervyn Maze over single-malt whiskey, his drink of choice, Pratik and I published our MENDS study in *JAMA*, proving that the standard practice of using benzos in ICU care was not the best or safest approach for treating critically ill patients. The MENDS patients had demonstrated that sledgehammer sedation was unnecessary. Once treated with a novel approach, they had suffered four fewer days with delirium and coma. To me, this provided great hope for ICU patients, a shifting of the needle toward a better hospital experience for patients, families, and health-care teams. We also suspected that it would translate into improved health in their lives after discharge.

Ultimately, the ABC trial was lauded by many who saw it as landmark proof that oversedation played a huge role in how long patients spent on the ventilator, in the ICU, and whether they lived or died. From the same patients, we learned that being awake on a ventilator did not increase psychological injury or accelerate mental health problems. While it was alarming and dispiriting to understand the magnitude of harm caused by the old way of care, it seemed as if we had found a real way forward. We would finally alter the trajectory of our patients' well-being, both in and after the ICU. I was delighted by the way these concrete data could be brought to the bedside to help patients maintain their brain health while we treated their critical illness.

The next steps for our ICU teams were to monitor our patients and hold them closer to the surface of consciousness without delirium, to give them only enough sedation to keep them comfortable for just long enough, then to let them stay awake, with their pain and anxiety handled with safer medications. Already some early-adopter nurses and doctors were beginning to change their approach, and my patients were starting to be awake and alert sooner after their ICU admission. I was hopeful that I would finally get to know them before we discharged them to other floors.

It was a long way from my first musings that the lung bone was connected to the brain bone. I wondered where we might head next.

• • •

Recently, I reread the notes I made as a young doctor caring for Teresa Martin more than three decades ago. Over the past few years, I had often thought about trying to find out what happened to her during her stay but had been reluctant. Perhaps I didn't want to know. Even when I decided to try, making multiple phone calls and sending dozens of emails to obtain permission, and received the cardboard box from North Carolina with its huge stack of notes, I hesitated before reading. Coming face-to-face with who you once were is always a little unnerving.

My nearly illegible handwriting was easy to recognize—it hasn't changed much over the years—spooling out in black pen across pages of lined paper, and I saw myself back then: eager, earnest, hungry. A young doctor wanting to master a rapidly developing field and to make a difference in people's lives. I had written the date at the top of the page like a promise: "8/26/89." Not yet knowing that the care I was about to provide would both save and ruin my young patient's life.

As I read through the notes, quickly at first and then settling in with them, I saw how oblivious I was at the time. How tipsy with confidence that technology would save the day. I noted with surprise that Teresa had a young son, something I hadn't known at the time. Or had known but dismissed as irrelevant to her medical care. By my own hand, Teresa Martin stayed on the ventilator for over sixty days, receiving breaths of air that were standard practice at the time to prevent lung collapse, but which I now knew were too large to fit inside her chest. This practice actually increased the likelihood of her dying. No wonder her lungs burst six times.

For the first thirty days, according to my notes, she was paralyzed and in a coma, receiving over 125 mg a day of both a benzodiazepine and morphine. A huge amount of a powerful sedative and an opioid shooting through her blood and infiltrating her brain. For the next thirty days, she stayed in bed, and after that she struggled to sit upright in a chair. I knew the notes wouldn't have any reference to delirium, and as I read, I found only recurrent mentions of her having ICU psychosis, to which I had attached the words "as expected." This made me heart-sick. At the time I thought of this as benign and had treated it with huge doses of the antipsychotic drug haloperidol. And then I had written a remarkably callow sentence: "However, amazingly enough, the patient still manifests only single organ damage (lungs) with good renal, GI, and cardiovascular function." How naive I was. And how far from the truth, as I would see a few weeks later when Teresa returned to me with her body and her brain irretrievably broken.

As physicians, we generally think we are most likely to harm our patients with an errant scalpel, a central line placement gone awry, or a medication error, but sometimes we cause more harm by blindly accepting usual practice as best practice. Familiarity can breed complacency. I believe this happened in critical care. Robert Jay Lifton, psychiatrist and author, coined the term *malignant normality*. He came to the idea after studying Nazi doctors and the normalcy of their extreme behavior within the structure of their world. We critical care doctors did not set out to cause harm. Within the ebb and flow of progress in science and medicine, we introduced new treatments and approaches to patient care in the hope of doing good, but sometimes we wrought harm instead. Indirectly and unintentionally, we caused enormous suffering by not questioning our practices, or by assuming that we could decide that the greater good of saving lives outweighed the side effects. It turned out that in some patients those side effects were, in large part, preventable.

Chapter 9

Awakening Change—Patients Are Resurfacing

> *Believe that a further shore*
> *Is reachable from here.*
> *Believe in miracles*
> *And cures and healing wells.*

> —Seamus Heaney, *The Cure at Troy*

IN MARCH OF 2012, I stood outside a daffodil-yellow cottage with a red-tiled roof on a cobblestone street in Odense, Denmark, a hundred miles west of Copenhagen. Two centuries earlier, this quaint building had been the childhood home of writer Hans Christian Andersen, and as I peered through the windows, I wondered if I might be about to encounter my own modern-day fairy tale. Earlier I had read a paper in the *Lancet* about a group of Danish physicians using a "no sedation" protocol in their ICU patients on ventilators, and I was determined to learn if it could possibly be true. I recalled that this small Scandinavian country had played a key role in the innovation of critical care before, pushing the field forward during the 1950s polio epidemics and the incipience of mechanical ventilation in the 1960s. But still, no sedation at all seemed extreme. I was prepared to expose it as a fallacy, much like the creation of the woven garments in Andersen's "The Emperor's New Clothes."

Dr. Palle Toft and Dr. Thomas Strøm met me at the bright red doors to the ICU at Odense University Hospital. Dr. Toft was an intensivist in charge of research operations there, and Dr. Strøm was the suddenly well-known doctor who was the lead author on the paper. He looked young, boyish with his jovial smile and dimpled cheeks, and wore sky-blue scrubs underneath his lab jacket.

"Welcome, Wes," said Dr. Toft, nodding. Perfectly coiffed and dressed in a wool suit and tie, he was smiling, too.

I was beginning to feel less adversarial already.

"Thank you for traveling all this way to our small country," said Dr. Strøm in flawless English. "Showing you our ICU and something of the lives of our patients is an honor."

I followed him through the doors and immediately saw a spacious room with the sun shining through sheer drapes onto a patient's face. He was sitting up in bed, next to the huge windows, flooded in light. It was as if the team were telling the patient, "Look out there, it's where you belong. Remember, this illness is only temporary!" As I drew closer, I could see that he was receiving ventilated breaths through an endotracheal tube, that he was surrounded by the usual trappings of ICU care, but there he was, alert and awake, a nurse standing over his right shoulder talking to him, and a physical therapist at the foot of the bed. The patient held a folder in his hands that looked like a menu. I thought he was choosing his lunch, but then he started to write. Dr. Strøm saw me tilt my head. "It's his *dagbog*, his diary. All of our patients and families use them to log what happens to them." I nodded. I'd read about Dr. Christina Jones, a PhD nurse in the UK who was a pioneer of the ICU diary, a tool we'd been too slow to adopt in the United States. I made a mental note. I had a feeling I'd be making many more over the next few hours.

In another room I saw a familiar sight, a daughter sitting at her mother's bedside, but in this case, they were holding hands and watching TV together, engrossed in a show. In our ICU rooms, it was usually family members who enjoyed the TV while the patients were either unconscious or staring blankly.

"Mrs. Damgaard is here for pneumococcal sepsis and ARDS," Dr. Strøm said. "Notice she's wide-awake on her vent and not on any sedation, even though she's still requiring seventy percent oxygen and a PEEP of twelve. Right, Mrs. Damgaard?" He turned to face her and said something in Danish, then explained to me she would be on the ventilator at least one more day.

Next Dr. Strøm led me into another sun-filled room, and I looked on as he joked around with a bald man wearing oversize glasses. I took in his indented temples and barrel-shaped chest, signs of emphysema. He was on ventilatory support with 65 percent oxygen, but again he was totally awake and alert. He proudly showed us a picture of his wife.

I knew that each patient here received several hours of deep sedation when the ventilator was initially started, but beyond that the practice deviated sharply from ours: patients received only small doses of morphine for any pain or discomfort they might feel, whereas our patients still received ongoing sedation that often left them unconscious for days into their ICU stay. Dr. Strøm and the team had received criticism that no sedation would lead to anxiety disorders and other mental health problems for their patients. We had heard similar negative feedback around our light sedation investigation, the ABC study, and had already disproved the theory. Patients seemed better able to handle their fears when they could see and understand what was happening to them. Later, when they were discharged, they were more equipped to process events when they weren't just fuzzy memories misinterpreted through a fog of delirium.

I continued with my tour. Room after room it was the same: intubated patients sitting up in beds with crisp striped sheets, communicating with their nurses and doctors through hand gestures and messages on dry-erase boards. And the nurses and doctors were responding, talking, smiling, and laughing. I stood and stared. There was so much activity. I watched nurses make plans with their patients about getting out of bed, deftly moving lines and tubes out of the way so they could help scoot their patient's legs to the side, and I saw patients walking with a physical therapist, the ventilator trailing behind them. This was what a protocol of no sedation—or perhaps more accurately called very light sedation—could achieve. Patients who were upright and mobile and involved in their own care, some within a day of arriving in the ICU. It was hard to equate that they were still critically ill even while they were fully awake and moving around. But they were. I had been focused on lowering sedation to save my patients' brains from injury, but now I saw that the natural extension was for them to be out of bed, then walking, then marching out of the ICU and back into their lives. It seemed that in this case the famed fairy-tale idiom was untrue: the emperor *did* have clothes on.

Later in my stay, I left the small town and went to bustling Copenhagen, past the brightly colored town houses of the city center and along the harbor to see the famous bronze statue memorializing one of Andersen's most beloved characters, the Little Mermaid. Unveiled on August 23, 1913, she gazes toward the Baltic Sea, a young woman who gave up her voice to exchange her mermaid tail for legs in pursuit of love and human connection. While Andersen's original fairy story does not conclude well for her, the modern version ends with the mermaid reclaiming her voice, gaining legs, and embarking on a new life beyond the ocean. As I stood looking out across the water, I laughed. I was thinking of Dr. Strøm's patients, who had swum out of the sea of sedation and found their voice and legs, too. But there was something else. A palpable current of kindness ran between the health-care team and their patients. It felt as though this had been hidden to me before, but now I saw that it was possible. I wanted to embrace it, too.

• • •

Since my mother's summer book club, I had loved reading Steinbeck, inspired by his empathy for the underdog. In his magnum opus, *East of Eden*, there's a passage that describes the exhilaration of being alive and how that joy colors the world with promise: "Sometimes a kind of glory lights up the mind of a man. It happens to nearly everyone. You can feel it growing or preparing like a fuse burning toward dynamite. It is a feeling in the stomach, a delight of the nerves, of the forearms. The skin tastes the air, and every deep-drawn breath is sweet." That was how I felt after Odense.

I returned home to Nashville with a sense of excitement and urgency, and also a freedom I had never before felt. I didn't have to practice medicine in the same old way. As our girls finished up their homework, I talked with Kim, walking with her through the soft dark of our neighborhood. I heard the enthusiasm in my voice. I could hardly wait to get back to the hospital. In my mind, I was already seeing my patients out of their beds and walking the wards just days after being admitted to the ICU.

"How will you do it?" she asked.

Kim knew just as I did that it would be extremely difficult to achieve, even in my ICU units, let alone farther afield. The forces that press against us in medicine to maintain the status quo are immense. It had already been difficult to convince people that our wake-up-and-breathe protocol was best for patients and to get our ICU teams on board. Every day on rounds, I would be surrounded by nurses, interns, residents, fellows, pharmacists, respiratory therapists, physical therapists, occupational therapists, palliative care, nutritionists, and social workers, a team of capable professionals, all of whom had been trained in a certain way to care for the sickest ICU patients. No sedation and early mobility went against everything they had ever learned. Even if I was able to make changes for a few patients under my direct care, the moment I was off service, things would likely revert to the status quo.

I could also see that we had to aim for more than local change. Even in Denmark, while patients flourished under the care of Dr. Strøm and his team, most of the other ICUs in the small country still sedated their patients, some quite heavily. Those of us sensing the need to transform care had to think globally. It was essential to reach the tens of thousands of ICU teams rounding every morning all over the world and be a part of their key decision-making for patients' treatment plans.

"The entire culture has to change. Starting with me. I have to do better." As I said it, I felt both oriented and lost. I knew what I wanted to do. I also knew everything the critical care community would need to accomplish to get there. It was big. The entire team in every ICU would have to be won over, comprising a health-care army of sorts, because it wasn't something any one doctor could achieve alone. I was reminded of a quote by author, theologian, and civil rights leader Howard Thurman: "There are two questions that we have to ask ourselves. The first is 'Where am I going?' and the second is 'Who will go with me?' If you ever get these questions in the wrong order, you are in trouble."

"I'll find others who will help," I said.

Kim nodded. "I'm sure you will. It's just going to take some time." She always had my back.

I knew other pioneers were out there. Just the month before, Dr. Dale Needham, an intensivist at Johns Hopkins, and Dr. Judy Davidson, a doctor of nursing practice from Scripps, published a paper with a panel of twenty-eight other ICU clinical-outcomes specialists, aimed at improving treatment for intensive care survivors. They had coined the term *post-intensive care syndrome* (PICS) to refer to a grouping of three long-term problems experienced by some survivors of critical illness including cognitive (brain dysfunction), mental health (depression, anxiety, and PTSD), and physical (muscle weakness and nerve damage) disabilities. Just like the problems of the people who had been finding their way to me after their hospital stays. I made a note to read the article again. I remembered browsing other recent papers on getting ventilated patients out of bed, on muscle wastage in the ICU, but at the time they had seemed like disembodied words on paper. My focus had been on delirium and sedation. Now their authors' names swam into my head: Polly Bailey, Dr. Richard Griffiths, Dr. Margaret Herridge, and Dr. Bill Schweickert. I recalled Dr. Herridge's recent groundbreaking work with ARDS patients showing that, five years after critical illness, survivors had difficulty functioning due to ICU-acquired weakness. I remembered Dr. Schweickert's landmark study on walking ventilated patients.

I had actually met him at the University of Chicago years before when he was designing his study on early mobility. My friends and his mentors, Dr. J. P. Kress and Dr. Jesse Hall, had laughed, saying, "We can't get him to calm down about this project." Eventually, he and his physical therapists started getting the intervention patients out of bed and mobile just a day and a half into their ICU ventilator experience, compared with the control patients, who started mobility after a week on average. It was a dramatic shift from usual care. This seminal investigation of just 104 patients helped the intervention patients regain strength and coordination and, surprisingly, cut the time they spent in delirium in half. This astonishing advance tripled a patient's odds of returning to physical independence by hospital discharge. It also, I thought, opened the door to them having less cognitive impairment after their ICU stay.

Yet, I wasn't sure that anything had changed in day-to-day critical care in response to the study. I was beginning to understand that seeing was believing. Everyone needed to have their Odense epiphany.

• • •

First, I had more questions for my friends in Denmark. My short stay there had so captivated me that I'd left without knowing key pieces of information needed to build a similar way forward. My thought was if I could learn their story, then I would be able to replicate it to convince others of the transformation we needed in critical care.

Dr. Toft was happy to fill me in. He explained that as a young intensivist at Odense in the late 1980s, he had used sedation rampantly, just like everywhere else in the world. Then, in 2003, after time away at a different hospital in Denmark, he returned to Odense to become a professor there and discovered that things had changed. "I was stunned to find that all the patients were—well, not all of them, ninety percent of the patients—were nonsedated." I laughed. I could well imagine his astonishment. During his time away, two rebel upstarts, Dr. Poul Klint Andersen and Dr. Søren Jepsen, had begun a mini-revolution.

I was curious to find out what had prompted Drs. Andersen and Jepsen to swim upstream against such a powerful current. Dr. Strøm took up the story. "They had several patients where they came to realize, 'Oh, there's a gargantuan mountain of sedation to overcome. It's a devil in our ICU.' So much midazolam had been accumulating in patients, they felt things were getting out of hand. And these patients looked so close to death they were about to consider withdrawing support and letting them die. When the patient eventually woke up, it was like, 'Oh, Jesus, what are we doing?'"

I was shocked. They had stopped sedation not because of a hunch that it might be negatively affecting their patients' outcomes, but due to guilt and fear. They had thought about removing life support because they believed their patients were already too far gone, too cognitively impaired. Just as Dr. Cook's *New England Journal of Medicine* paper had shown: the most modifiable reason for removing life support was a physician's guesstimate that long-term cognitive impairment was likely. But when they had seen patients wake up and recover against those odds, it scared them into radical change.

"But surely you had some resistance?" I asked. "From nurses maybe?" One of our veteran nurses had told me she went into critical care precisely because the patients were still most of the day and night. Dr. Strøm agreed that it had been difficult at first, but over time things had changed. A few years earlier, several nurses had come to the Odense ICU from one with a culture of deep sedation, and they had rejoiced at the opportunity to have more intimate and thorough human interactions. One said, "Oh, wow, I'm a nurse again."

It made sense that the nurses appreciated the increased connection with the patients and having a proper role in their care. This would be key. Would seeing the change in patients such as these bring others on board? It had certainly sold me. My mind raced to our not having one-to-one nursing in the United States. Most ICUs around the world assign two patients to every nurse, so called two to one, and some countries have even higher ratios. We would have to work with this somehow.

I still didn't understand something. If no sedation was going so well in Odense, how and why was a clinical trial ever conducted? Dr. Toft piped up, "That was me. Obviously, the idea to stop sedating was Poul's and Søren's, but it was my idea to say, 'We need to do science about this. We need to prove it, otherwise nobody else will believe us, and we'll be just one center in the world doing this.'"

I was reminded of what my mentor Dr. Haponik had always taught me: "If you don't write it up, it never happened." Dr. Toft was in the strange position of having to test no sedation against sedation, so he had to intervene with an *increase* in sedation for the trial. I asked what happened when they first told others about their data. I knew there was a lot of disbelief when the paper was published. I had been one of the doubters myself. I had heard about a grand rounds lecture Dr. Strøm presented in Pittsburgh in which he gave a preview of what he was submitting to the *Lancet*. "That was terrible," he said, laughing. "They said, 'Okay, we're having a hard time following. This guy is saying no sedation. That's like the Wild West.' I showed them more results, and they looked at it very politely, but I could see they were thinking, 'This guy is just crazy. Is he really a doctor?' They said, 'It's like a fairy tale and we don't believe it.'"

• • •

Recently I described my visit to the Odense ICU to a friend and she said, "It sounds like the movie *Awakenings*." In the film, based on neurologist Oliver Sacks's book of the same name, Robin Williams plays a fictional Dr. Sacks, and Robert De Niro is his catatonic patient Leonard Lowe. Watching Leonard—and then the other patients—come back to life after decades of living closed away from the world around them is extraordinary. While my experience in the Danish ICU was quite different, there were resounding similarities. The movie has a sense of wonder, and of possibility, that I had witnessed in Odense, too. A realization that human connection is everything. At the beginning, the hospital ward where the catatonic patients live is referred to by the staff as "the garden" because the patients there are simply to be fed and watered. But by the end, a shift has occurred, and the patients are cared for as humans. In a powerful moment, Williams addresses a group of hospital donors: "The human spirit is more powerful than any drug, and that is what needs to be nourished, with work, play, friendship, family. These are the things that matter. This is what we'd forgotten. The simplest things." Not only are the patients awakened—though briefly—but the doctors and nurses, too. In Odense, I had experienced my own awakening.

I was driven by science to help patients, assiduously designing trials and answering questions, determined to make a difference in critical care. Finally in Odense I had put it all together: follow the science and find the humanity. Recently I read this quote by writer Rebecca Solnit: "Scientists too, as J. Robert Oppenheimer once remarked, 'live always at the "edge of mystery"—the boundary of the unknown.' But they transform the unknown into the known, haul it in like fishermen; artists get you out into that dark sea." I liked to think that physicians did both.

After Odense, I consciously decided to consider disease only with the entire person in my focus. It may have seemed obvious, and I may even have thought that I was already treating patients in this manner, but in reality I was still holding back. Purposely so. I had moved forward from what I was taught during training: to steel myself against emotions and connection. But I was still only partially meeting my patients where they were. I empathized at the bedside and treated them to the best of my technical ability, but a world was still between us: patient and physician. I was taking care of them, which suggests handling or managing, rather than caring for them. Sedation solidified this distance.

In the months after my trip to Denmark, I decided I was ready to plunge in. I was willing to "enter into the chaos of another," as bioethicist and theologian James F. Keenan says in defining mercy. I decided it was a somewhat incomplete definition, however, because I'd been diving into the chaos of the ICU for years without necessarily providing lifting and healing. Whether by corporal acts or by spiritual gestures and conversations, guided always by the patient's wishes, I wanted to achieve a more universal form of healing, especially when cure was not possible. It would come at a cost, and I knew that. Time, relationships with colleagues, and personal tranquility were at stake.

Every day, I made sure that my first action with my patient was to make eye contact, to touch her gently to be certain she knew I saw her, and she saw me. Then one by one, I tried to find out something new about each person. Something that didn't directly relate to her illness. I strove to remember that each patient carried his own life story into the ICU, his own narrative that did not stop once he was under my watch. That brought me into the right relationship with my patients, which improved my care. I noticed that at times I walked away from patients' beds feeling a viselike grip around my chest, a sense of hurt, and I understood it came from feeling mercy. Derived from the Latin *misericordia*, mercy indicates the suffering of the heart, or compassion—*cum patior* (I suffer with). The *with* brought me back to *empathy*, meaning "to feel with." Compassion can be understood as empathy in action. I had long been a believer in researcher and bioethicist Dr. Jodi Halpern's work on clinical empathy, especially her teaching that compassion should never be an extra step in our care, but an adverb to describe *how* we care. Now I began to feel comfortable putting it into practice. I had needed to work my way toward it. I found that connecting with patients, opening myself up to them, took me no more time in a day, and the pressure I felt deep in my chest told me I was being a physician, a healer for my patients, and not just a "provider." I was out in that dark sea, finding my way.

• • •

In July 1994, in Kaysville, Utah, just a few miles east of the Great Salt Lake, Joy Sundloff developed septic shock during a routine gallbladder surgery and was rushed by helicopter to the ICU at LDS Hospital. There, nurse Polly Bailey recognized Joy's name—she knew exactly who in their small town did Joy's hair and nails—and took her under her wing as her patient. For the next fifty days Polly looked after Joy in the hospital, attending to her needs as she lay comatose on a ventilator, updating Joy's husband, John, at every opportunity. Polly was the nurse who oversaw Joy when she finally made it out of the ICU and into the rehab unit. When Joy returned home to Kaysville, Polly made daily visits to the house where Joy lived with John and their two young children.

Last year I went to Utah to meet with Polly, Joy, and John and talk about their experience with ICU care. I hadn't known them at the time of Joy's hospitalization—I was still a pulmonology and critical care fellow at Wake Forest—but I had met Polly about eight years ago in Salt Lake City when I was figuring out how to get my patients upright and out of bed, and to spread the word about it. She was one of the innovators. At our first meeting, she told me that when she opened up *JAMA* in 2004 and read my delirium mortality paper, she had started crying. Hearing that meant so much to me, knowing how many late nights and early mornings I had channeled into the study. "I knew that finally we would have data to support what had happened to Joy," Polly said.

Joy and John had invited me over, along with Polly, and some other ICU team members, and we were diving into a delicious homemade brunch: a sausage-and-egg casserole, a stack of waffles oozing syrup, and platters of fruit salad. Though Joy's ICU stay had happened decades before, its shadow was still in the room, binding them tightly to one another. When Polly visited Joy's home all those years earlier, it was the first time Polly had seen a patient beyond the walls of the ICU. She was shocked by what she witnessed. Joy couldn't get out of bed herself as her muscles had wasted away. Fifty days paralyzed in a bed would do that. Her muscle loss wasn't visible at first because of all the fluids she had been given to keep her blood pressure up and her heart pumping. "She gained fifty pounds of water weight in what they called a third space," said John. But the results of the muscle wasting were obvious. Even with help, it took Joy four hours to shower. John had quit work to care for her. Getting downstairs—which she did just once a day—took the support of an army of helpers from her local church community. Playing with her children was out of the question, and getting her hair and nails done couldn't have been further from her mind. She could barely string a sentence together. The words she needed rolled through her mind, but she couldn't catch them quickly enough for them to make sense. She wanted to go back to coordinating a community youth group, but she didn't know where to start. Joy's life was in ruins. She had post-intensive care syndrome—though she didn't know it. She was thirty-six years old.

Polly's astonishment and outrage had taken her to her boss, Dr. Terry Clemmer, a classically trained physiologist and pulmonologist. She described him as the kind of doctor who sat with patients all night, watching over the machines, trying to figure out what to do next to save someone's life. As she said this, I was thinking back to the way I had looked after my own early patients, my eyes on the monitors, my focus on the lungs. And all the while, the patient was being harmed without my knowledge and then would go home and live a ruined life that I had no idea about.

"I saw what happened to Joy," said Polly, "and that changed everything. I knew that we had caused it. I said to Terry, 'I'm going to fix this process. . . . We're just going to change everything.' He said, 'Okay, you bring me the literature.' So I took him a stack of papers a foot high and said, 'Here you go. But there's nothing in there to support what we're going to do.'" Polly paused and took a sip of orange juice. "There wasn't literature about delirium, there wasn't literature about weaning sedation. There wasn't literature about mobility, there wasn't literature about anything."

Even now, she had fire in her eyes as she spoke. "I told Terry that if we had patients strong, if we started activity, they would come off the ventilator faster. But he said, 'Activity has nothing to do with getting a patient extubated.'"

I knew exactly what Dr. Clemmer had been thinking. We all thought the same thing back then: that we were trying to fix the lung, and how could activity possibly help with that? We should have been thinking, as Polly was, that the lungs are surrounded by rib cage muscles and the diaphragm, which need exercise, and that without it—especially if a patient is lying in a coma—they will grow weak. Polly shook her finger in my face. "I said, 'You are absolutely wrong, Terry Clemmer!'—with my finger wagging just like this. I was mad." She laughed. "Later he came to me and said, 'Okay, what is it that you want to do?'"

She revolutionized care in her ICU by bringing in physical therapists to improve patients' muscle strength, and to teach the nurses how to get the patients out of bed earlier. It made a remarkable difference for the patients she oversaw. But Polly wanted more than an early-mobility innovation. Her mind-set enabled her to see the patients' point of view. She had decided to become a nurse as a young girl, and her empathy and caring showed. They had been strong enough to make her take action.

One of the things that struck me most about Joy's story was the way the unintentional harm caused by sedation and lack of mobility manifested in seemingly tiny ways yet were momentous to her experience as a patient. One evening, bed bound with profound muscle damage, she managed to summon the strength to inch her arm high enough to reach the call light next to her bed and to press it. When the nurse's voice responded, asking what she needed, Joy was unable to answer because she was intubated. The nurse never came to assist her. The thought of her lying there alone, in need, pained me. That happened over twenty-five years ago. I like to think we've made some strides since then.

• • •

One of my most vivid memories of visiting the ICU in Odense was of a critically ill patient walking slowly with her physical therapist, her ventilator trailing behind like a small and faithful dog. It was such a perfect adaptation of technology. We did this in our ICU, too, but never so early—we always waited until a patient's critical illness had quiesced. I realized that Odense was so different because all these innovations were completely routine there. That's what I was hoping we could achieve. It seemed to me that, in addition to nurses, physical therapists were pivotal to bring on board, as they were specifically trained in biomechanics and would surely make the connection between early activity and better physical outcomes.

After my visit to Denmark, I attended a conference in Houston and noticed a talk on early ICU mobility on the roster. It sounded perfect. It was to be given by Christiane "Chris" Perme, a physical therapist and board-certified cardiovascular and pulmonary clinical specialist at Houston Methodist Hospital. I squeezed into the back of a packed hall and listened to Chris speak with confidence and charisma about her considerable experience in working with ventilated patients. She talked about the challenging atmosphere of physical therapy in the ICU, with patients who were so close to death and often hooked up to many lines and machines. But then she described her methods and made me see it was doable, even on a larger scale than in Odense. She reeled off a long list of possible positive outcomes when ICU patients undertake guided exercise and walking programs: better cardiopulmonary and neuromuscular function, greater independence, improved patient attitude, earlier ventilator liberation, decreased length of hospital stay and costs, and high level of satisfaction for nurses, patients, physicians, therapists, and family members. This last one made a strong impression on me. It was what Thomas Strøm had said about their nurses. Getting patients awake and moving meant more hard work, but patient connection and personal satisfaction might make all the difference.

Chris and I have become good friends over the years, and recently I invited her to Vanderbilt to give a lecture to our ICU teams. I asked her why she decided to become a physical therapist in the first place. Her epiphany occurred at her high school's career day in the small town of Ribeirão Preto, São Paulo, Brazil. At that time she was Christiane de Souza Strambi. "I was sitting in a gym, sixteen years old, when a woman came onstage and told us her job was to help people walk again. I started dreaming right then about getting people vertical." Chris went home and told her mother she was going to be a *fisioterapeuta*. The career just seemed to speak to her. Later, she received a degree in physical therapy from Pontifical Catholic University of Campinas, but to pursue her dream further, she decided to move to the United States. With her fiancé, Dario, she obtained visas and secured floor space on a rickety cargo ship that, once at sea, soon lost all communication with the outside world due to a broken radio. After three weeks of being rocked by storms and veering well off course, they finally reached New Orleans in 1985.

At the time, I was just a few city blocks away, finishing up my final semester of college and getting ready to start medical school. It was a small world. Eventually Chris's training led her to critical care medicine and Houston, where Dr. Jorge Mario Gonzalez, a pulmonologist, asked her to get patients on ventilators out of bed and walking. Chris was terrified. She said to the doctor, "But they're attached to that machine. Nobody can walk on that." I nodded. It was astonishing to me that Dr.

Gonzalez had even suggested it, in 1994, the same year Joy Sundloff had landed in the ICU. And just like Polly Bailey, Chris was surprised to find a dearth of medical literature. "There was nothing written on the subject," said Chris.

At first, she hesitated. She was scared she'd harm her patients. Then one day she noticed a patient being transported from the ICU to radiology for a scan. "They brought a shoebox-type thing and hooked her up, and I asked what it was. 'Well, that's a Hamilton portable ventilator.' At that time the vent we had was huge, the size of a go-cart."

The next time Dr. Gonzalez approached her about a patient he wanted to see walking, she described the Hamilton used by the respiratory department. Immediately, Gonzalez picked up the phone and called the director of respiratory care. "Chris Perme says there's a ventilator in this hospital that is a little blue box. I want that ventilator here in five minutes." When it arrived, Gonzalez said, "Now you hook that up to your patient and get them up and walking." With the doctor at her side, Chris helped the patient out of bed, swinging her legs around slowly, then lowering her onto her feet. As she described the scene, I pictured it. I had watched it many times by then, those first tentative steps, the light that goes on in a patient's eyes as they acknowledge that they can do this. That they are walking. Even while critically ill and still attached to the ventilator. It's a huge step—both literally and figuratively.

In the beginning, Chris was still convinced that her patients would fall and hurt themselves and possibly die—after all, they were gravely ill. She admitted, "Many times I would go to the bathroom to cry and cry and cry. I was so nervous." But one day an elderly patient, Teresa Hernandez, was admitted and placed on a ventilator due to severe pneumonia. Before her hospital stay, she had lived an independent life in the house where she had raised her children. Although polio had paralyzed her right leg years earlier, she stayed active, walking and climbing stairs using a leg brace. Once on the ventilator, Teresa grew steadily weaker, and it seemed unlikely that she would ever have the strength she needed to be weaned from the machine and breathe on her own again. The likelihood of her returning to her home was slim. Dr. Gonzalez looked at Chris and said, "If you do not make her walk, she's going to die. But if you get her up, she's going to live. It's that simple."

Chris was determined to get Teresa moving, to restore her muscles, and to help her wean off the ventilator so that she could live in her own home again. Day by day, Chris helped Teresa regain her strength, until eventually she was able to leave the ICU and head home, ventilator-free, and walking with a cane. Chris had found her calling as a physical therapist in critical care, advocating for early walking and activity for ICU patients, and eventually writing papers and further spreading the word. She never looked back.

I found Polly's and Chris's stories captivating. They were both inspired to do what was right for their patients by seeing how a hospital stay affected a patient out in the world. Knowing that a patient will likely be discharged to her own home instead of a nursing home or even instead of dying in the hospital is a powerful motivator. I was struck again by the need to change the way we designate success in the ICU. We need to listen to what our patients want and help them achieve it.

• • •

On rereading Steinbeck's *East of Eden*, first published in 1952, I was astonished to find an accurate depiction of the physical effects of PICS, the damage done to nerves and muscles through prolonged bed rest. "When I recovered from my pneumonia it came time for me to learn to walk again. I had been nine weeks in bed, and the muscles had gone lax and the laziness of recovery had set in. When I was helped up, every nerve cried, and the wound in my side, which had been opened to drain the pus from the pleural cavity, pained horribly. I fell back in bed, crying, 'I can't do it! I can't get up!'" In just a few sentences, Steinbeck describes the devastation of the body after serious illness, the need for rehabilitation, and the patient's emotional pain, sixty years before the term PICS was coined.

After Odense, I was curious to know exactly what happened to a patient's body when he stayed in bed, motionless, for days on end. I had seen the effects of this wasting in patients' lives, but what did it look like inside the body? I had run into a British doctor, Richard Griffiths, at various conferences, and one of his classic papers on muscle atrophy in critical care had been in my peripheral vision. He was always fun to talk to, cheerful and erudite, and I set about reading his work. He showed that the skeletal muscles of critically ill and immobilized patients are used by their body as a protein source to fight the illness, in much the same way that endurance athletes burn muscle and fat when their body runs out of calories. In this case, though, the loss of muscle mass was extreme. While this wasting could be mitigated to some extent by tube feedings, Dr. Griffiths showed that the burning process was still ablaze. Only once the patient moved again did the body begin to replenish that store of muscle.

His work had helped reveal that for every day spent inactive in the ICU, two or more weeks of activity were needed to rebuild that muscle. It was astonishing to me that I hadn't known this, that few of us in critical care were aware of this. We were leaving our patients dormant in the bed for far too long in the name of safety. Other areas of medicine, too, were complicit in creating inadvertent harm: from treating patients with tuberculosis in sanatoriums, to recommending bed rest for patients with blood clots in their legs, as well as after childbirth. I found it so frustrating. It seemed to be a perennial problem that the outcomes of our treatments were only discovered once the patients were long gone from our care.

· · ·

A few months ago, I reconnected with Dr. Griffiths. He was in Provence, France, where he lives part of the year, having retired from an illustrious career at Whiston Hospital near Liverpool, the site of one of the first ICUs in England. He was raised in north London, his father in charge of the Chartered Institute of Transport and his mother a biology teacher. I asked him about his education. "I grew up knowing plants, animals, and everything. I went to medical school in 1971 at University College in central London, and during my third year, I did a separate degree in muscle physiology and later worked with two Nobel laureates, Bernard Katz and Sir Andrew Huxley." Huxley won the Nobel Prize for sodium transport along the nerves and later introduced the sliding filament hypothesis of muscles, an explanation of how muscles contract that has remained the basis of modern understanding of muscle physiology. Thus, Dr. Griffiths came by his knowledge of the neuromuscular system honestly.

"I studied the way nerves meet and communicate with one another and then tell the muscles when and how long to contract." Dr. Griffiths spoke quickly, hands flying up and down. I remembered that feeling of his being three thoughts ahead and trying to catch up.

Through a tangled web of jobs over the next decade, Dr. Griffiths became a pediatrician, then a neonatologist, and then stumbled into a research position where he biopsied muscles. He had never set foot in an ICU when, in 1985, he was hired as a consultant in Dr. Eric Sherwood-Jones's ICU at Whiston Hospital. Sherwood was a pioneer of intensive care medicine in the UK. Dr. Griffiths laughed. "They said to me, 'You know a lot about medicine that we don't know. We can teach you all about adult intensive care, the things that *we* know.'"

When he started his work there, he had never seen a patient paralyzed and sedated on a ventilator before and was horrified by what seemed to be an aggressive approach to illness. As he spoke, I was thinking how bed after bed of comatose patients must be a shocking sight if it's not something you encounter every day.

Many of the patients admitted to Whiston back then came in with flail chests from car accidents as people were still fairly lax about wearing seat belts. They usually sustained broken ribs and lung damage from hitting the steering wheel and ended up on ventilators for a week or ten days. Dr. Griffiths had an idea. "I had these patients coming in with flail chest, but their legs were all right. They were being paralyzed for seven days, so therefore they were immobilized. I could take one leg and mobilize it, using passive motion devices several hours a day. The other leg was the internal control." In this way, he undertook an interventional study to understand the effects of immobilization on muscle loss, and the effects of passive exercise on muscles. When he took muscle biopsies, he found that the immobilized leg had profound muscle degeneration, while passive stretch reduced protein loss and caused less muscle fiber wasting. "So I told them," Dr. Griffiths said, "'We can't leave these people immobilized. It's creating a new disease!'" He added, "The muscle loss isn't visible at first because the weakened muscle remains swollen with fluid. It can be several weeks before the wasting becomes obvious."

I thought back to John Sundloff saying how bloated Joy was well after her ICU stay. According to Dr. Griffiths, it could take weeks for the edema to shift and the muscle loss to be measurable. When people finally looked in the mirror, they often wouldn't recognize themselves. But again, the ICU teams didn't see the patients once they were discharged from their care. It was a secret disaster, one hiding in plain sight for decades.

It's little wonder that Joy Sundloff couldn't walk without help after spending fifty days strapped into an ICU bed on a ventilator. Or that thanks to physical therapy, Teresa Hernandez walked out of the hospital to return to independent living. Richard Griffiths's study provided the science to support Polly Bailey's and Chris Perme's work on the importance—and life-changing results—of early mobility in ICU patients.

When I had seen the patients in Odense awake and moving so early in their illness, I had focused on how good it was for them to see themselves as people again. It was beneficial for their souls. Yet, through Dr. Griffiths's work, I understood it was essential for their physical health, for their strength and mobility, and that would translate into their ability to reenter their post-ICU lives.

Human behavior is strange. Even though I had known about the work of these early mobility pioneers, had visited Polly Bailey in Salt Lake City, had heard about Bill Schweickert's landmark study on walking ventilated patients from his own lips, I still didn't register the magnitude of their findings until I went to Denmark and saw the fairy tale in action. Only then was I ready to accept the challenge and attempt to follow in their footsteps.

• • •

As I was leaving the ICU in Odense, Thomas Strøm glanced through one of the large windows at the red rooftops then turned to me.

"Our local writer Hans Christian Andersen was terrified of being buried alive. When he went to bed, he had a little note next to him saying, 'I'm not dead, I'm just sleeping.'"

Then Dr. Strøm laughed and so did I. Later, as I toured dozens of ICUs in many different countries, I came to realize that much good might come from signs above patients' beds that read, "I'm not dead, I'm just sedated."

Chapter 10

Spreading the Word—Putting New Ideas into Practice

What one man can do himself directly is but little. If however he can stir up ten others to take up the task he has accomplished much.

—Wilbur Wright, letter to Octave Chanute

ROB HARMER GREW UP on a farm in the tiny village of Fullarton, Ontario, racing dirt bikes and tearing apart carburetors. His parents encouraged him to get his hands dirty and to work hard. While school came easily, it wasn't a priority until a mentor at the local farm implement store, noting his intelligence, urged Rob to continue his education. And so he did, turning his intuitive understanding of engines and the way things worked into the study of mechanical engineering and, later, a job at a refinery, overseeing a group of research engineers. Rob was still an adventurous spirit, though, racing cars and motorbikes, and planning a trip to go skydiving and scuba diving in Australia when he met Bonnie McKay, a nurse. Drawn in by his gregarious nature and his good looks, Bonnie brought Rob to her sister's wedding.

That first date led to love, and they were married two years later, in 1994, and soon had their children, Lance and Kaely. Together they raised the kids, while he ascended the ranks as an executive in the chemical industry and she pursued nursing and teaching. Rob had a passion for troubleshooting problems and finding solutions and eventually held multiple patents, including one for solar panel technology. He still found time for family, chasing the kids around the house, coaching Lance's hockey teams, and hunkering down with Kaely as she worked on her math homework.

One day in 2005, Rob injured his elbow, and two days later it was red and swollen, and he was running a high fever. Bonnie insisted they go to their local hospital. Doctors there suspected cellulitis, a bacterial skin infection, and were amazed by its rapid progression throughout his body. Within hours, it looked as if his arm would have to be amputated. Suddenly Rob was fighting for his life. At only forty-three years old, he was rushed via ambulance to Detroit's Henry Ford Hospital, where he was diagnosed with sepsis and toxic shock syndrome. He had developed a rare skin and soft tissue infection called necrotizing fasciitis, better known as flesh-eating disease. The ICU team took extraordinary measures to save Rob's life and his arm, performing multiple operations to debride his wound and remove dead tissue destroyed by the infection. He spent three weeks on a ventilator as his body responded to treatments and eventually rallied. He struggled with delirium, thinking he was in a prison camp, that there was blood everywhere, or that Bonnie was plotting against him. But, as the nurses said, he was lucky to be alive, and when he headed home, he was ready to pick up life where he had left off. Kaely had made a duck sticker for him while he was sick, and he carefully moved it from the cast on his elbow to his wallet, a memory of his time in the hospital.

• • •

One chilly spring morning, I received an email from Dr. Lealani Acosta, a cognitive neurologist at Vanderbilt. "Dr. Ely, I have permission to consult with you about a new patient, Rob Harmer, who has me totally perplexed. He's a 52-year-old engineer who drove down here with his wife Bonnie to see me for a full dementia evaluation. They claim he got this from an ICU stay nine years ago in 2005, during which he experienced a lot of delirium. He said his life has been a 'downhill living hell' ever since. Imaging in the past showed no strokes. He's way too young to have dementia, has no comorbidities, normal labs, and I just can't explain my findings on exam or his neurocognitive tests. It's incongruous and unsettling. Is it possible that he got a dementia-like illness *de novo* from a single ICU stay?"

As I read, my stomach crawled with discomfort. It *was* incongruous and unsettling, but I thought the answer to her question was yes. I responded, suggesting a time to meet in person the following week. Communication via email was insufficient for the amount of nuanced information we had to sift through, and I had questions about the details of the ICU stay. Dr. Acosta assured me she would find out more before our meeting. Over the next few days, my mind returned to the email. While I had received others from distressed patients and families concerned about foggy thoughts or ongoing nightmares after a hospital stay, this was the first from a dementia expert. She was clearly bewildered by what she had seen in her patient. I had experienced that feeling many times myself.

Just one year earlier, we had definitively shown that people with no preexisting brain problems could emerge from critical illness with dementia. For years we had known a critical care stay could lead to some degree of cognitive impairment and had suspected something even more sinister. Finally, our NIH-sponsored BRAIN-ICU investigation had proved it. The study showed that during their critical care stay, more than one in three patients developed dementia that looked a lot like Alzheimer's disease and traumatic brain injury (TBI). It disrupted their day-to-day functioning and lasted at least one year. According to the study, the longer patients experienced delirium in the ICU, the more likely they were to develop dementia. While these findings were shocking in themselves, I was especially disturbed by the data showing it was occurring in people in their thirties, forties, and fifties. People such as Richard Langford, who was forced to retire early from his job as a minister, and Sarah Beth Miller.

I had never been able to shake the image of Sarah Beth's post-ICU brain, shrunken like a shriveled biceps when a cast is removed. A woman in her early fifties with the brain of a demented eighty-five-year-old. The memory had inspired me to set up a substudy of BRAIN-ICU with Dr. Jim Jackson and neuroscientist Dr. Ramona Hopkins, our colleague from Brigham Young University. This neuroimaging program, called VISIONS, enabled us to obtain and analyze brain MRIs of ICU survivors. We brought on board one of my mentees, a young Italian geriatrician named Alessandro Morandi, who threw himself into the project. A music lover, he had grown up in the town of Cremona, home of the Stradivarius, and in thickly accented English he urged the team on with "If the violin is out of tune, we must discover why!" Later, when I looked at the scans of the ICU survivors, the results were chilling. The brain dysfunction was writ large as the imaging revealed the same atrophy as seen on Sarah Beth's, and the survivors' extreme cognitive impairment and memory loss showed up as a reduction in the size of the hippocampus and the frontal cortex, regions of the brain that control neuropsychological tasks of memory and executive function.

No wonder these ICU survivors were unable to figure out the TV remote they had used for years or would forget they had already taken their medications. We had seen this over and over. A patient of mine had racked up over $1,000 in parking tickets because she could never remember where she had parked her car. Another patient almost lost his house because he kept forgetting to make his mortgage payments. The data showed the more severe a patient's delirium, the greater the atrophy in the hippocampus and the frontal cortex. I imagined that an MRI of Rob Harmer's brain would look the same.

A week later I was sitting in my office when my phone rang. It

158

was Dr. Acosta. "We don't need to meet. I just heard back from Bonnie Harmer." Dr. Acosta was crying. "Mr. Harmer took his own life." Everything stopped. I sank down into my chair. She kept talking, but I heard little of what she said. They were just words spinning in my ear. Dementia. Recovery. Gun. I didn't know what to say.

I left my office in a daze, stumbling into the elevator and out into the spring sunlight. All around me trees bloomed in a chorus of pink and purple, and everywhere I looked people seemed to be filled with joy. With purpose. Rob Harmer had lost his. His death shook me to the core as a physician, and as a husband and father. I felt saddened by the depths to which this illness had taken him, the way it had stolen hope. One minute he was playing with his kids, and the next, he couldn't envision any kind of future for himself. I had seen survivors struggling, trying to figure out how to live a different kind of life, but suicide? I shook my head. I could only imagine the pain that had led him down that path.

As I walked along, I was struck again by Dr. Acosta's confusion in the wake of Rob Harmer's symptoms, and I began to think about others with dementia and Alzheimer's. How many of them might have doctors who never connected an ICU stay with subsequent cognitive decline? How many of them, stuck in the fog of their demented thoughts, were also mired in their doctors' lack of knowledge about PICS? And how many of my own former patients might be out in the world somewhere, alone in an abyss of despair?

• • •

I hadn't known it at the time, but Bonnie Harmer was a nurse with two master's degrees and a PhD in education. She had seen delirium in patients in the wards, but more than that, she'd lived with it in her husband. She'd considered a connection between his many days of ICU delirium and his mental health and cognitive struggles since leaving Henry Ford. Eventually her curiosity had led her to reach out to Dr. Acosta at Vanderbilt.

When I tracked down Bonnie and we spoke, I was impressed by her desire to spread the word about PICS, to prevent others from going through the horror that Rob had experienced. At her nursing college, she passionately teaches students about delirium and PICS and instructs the new nurses how to use the CAM-ICU at the bedside. As she told me about Rob's critical illness and his treatment, I nodded. It felt like déjà vu. He had received the standard care of deep sedation and benzos. Plus an antipsychotic to treat his delirium. In 2005, I would have done exactly the same thing. I would have been relieved to have saved his life and sent him home to his family. Then I probably wouldn't have thought much about him as I turned my attention to the next patient on the gurney. Bonnie revealed that after his ICU discharge, Rob had suffered PTSD and an anxiety disorder that manifested as paranoia, nightmares, flashbacks, and insomnia. He also developed severe depression. A psychiatrist and other doctors prescribed a host of medications and several therapies including eye movement desensitization and reprocessing (EMDR), biofeedback, and counseling, but nothing had helped him.

As the years passed, Bonnie started to notice the cognitive decline. Her husband, a onetime math wizard and inventor, struggled to calculate simple problems such as 5 times 13 and could no longer help Kaely with her algebra. Bonnie recalled how much he had loved rebuilding Corvettes. He had done frame-off restorations, which meant stripping the car completely down and then rebuilding it. "He got to the point where he couldn't remember how to put the cars back together," she said, shaking her head at the memory. In my mind, I could see the parts of the car scattered everywhere, a jigsaw puzzle of frustration, one that mirrored Rob's life. He just couldn't get the pieces to fit.

After extensive neurocognitive testing, the Harmers were told what they probably already knew: that Rob was totally disabled with a dramatically slow processing speed for mental activities, and an inability to carry out the executive tasks that had made him so successful at work. I realized that Rob's problems were similar to chronic traumatic encephalopathy (CTE), a dementia that develops in many retired professional football players in their early forties.

Rob ended up taking a two-year disability leave to get the medical support he needed. Toward the end of that time, when he was preparing to return to his job, he began to feel encouraged. Bonnie's voice lifted: "He went from feeling total despair to finding hope again." She recalled the day the family went to Chicago to shop for some work clothes. Walking through the department store, Rob got sidetracked, as was common by this time, and decided to buy a fifteen-foot-long stainless-steel countertop that they didn't need. Bonnie remembered her confusion. Rob bought ratchet straps to tie it to the top of the car, then struggled. "This is a guy who grew up on a farm, a mechanical engineer, and he couldn't figure how to work the straps." Her voice sank. "It caused him a lot of irritation." I guessed that happened a lot. I wasn't sure if the countertop ever made it home with them. It wasn't the point of the story, but I imagined it in the parking lot, heaved off the car and discarded. Just one more reminder of a life gone askew.

After meeting with Dr. Acosta, Bonnie said they had felt there might be a way forward. There would be testing and at least an understanding of what had happened to Rob. A validation of sorts. They had made the trip home, planning to spend Mother's Day with Kaely and Lance. As they pulled into their driveway, they saw the front porch was filled with boxes. "Basically, they had emptied out his office, sent everything home, and told him that he was fired," Bonnie recounted. "When he saw that they weren't taking him back, it just crushed him."

I could see the sadness in her eyes. The next day was Rob Harmer's last.

While I wanted to avoid making assumptions, in talking to Bonnie a picture had emerged. Most people who seek to end their life due to illness are not looking for relief from pain or physical suffering. I knew this from extensive studies of people who pursue physician-assisted suicide and euthanasia. Instead, the number one reason is existential suffering. Suicide is complicated, and there isn't always a cause-and-effect relationship between a single event and the decision to end one's life, but in Rob's case it seemed as if a straight line could be drawn from his ICU stay filled with delirium to his development of progressive dementia and depression. He had told Bonnie, "My connections with people are sort of fading." I looked at photos of Rob that Bonnie shared. Grinning into the camera, his eyes wide, the future bright. A perfect family. A kiss with his wife in front of the Trevi Fountain in Rome. A T-shirt emblazoned with LIFE IS GOOD. I swallowed down a lump in my throat. When those boxes arrived on their doorstep unannounced, perhaps he saw his future as hopelessly compromised.

It didn't have to be that way.

• • •

After Rob Harmer's death, I tried to find some comfort in the knowledge that we were starting to make a difference for other patients. It had taken over fifteen years to gather the data that proved the old treatment of critical illness, including deep sedation and immobilization, was causing harm to the brain and the body, but now a consensus was growing, bolstered by mounting papers published in high-impact journals. While it would be unscientific to pin Rob Harmer's dementia on any one cause, the most likely preventable contributors were the enormous doses of benzodiazepines he received, and the prolonged delirium he suffered during his hospitalization for sepsis. We had learned since then that benzos were strong predictors of the development of delirium, which in turn was the strongest predictor of post-ICU dementia. By 2014, the year of Rob's death, in twenty-seven studies over twenty-five years in over three thousand ICU patients, not once were benzodiazepines found to be superior to any of the medications to which they were compared. Yet they were the most commonly used sedative in critical care. Following the science, we had started to take a different path, one that when put into practice was already beginning to change the lives of our critically ill patients. Physicians such as me and many others in health care were leading the charge to prevent or lessen the damage caused to the brain and body during an ICU stay, and the focus of others lay in supporting patients after discharge. We had the ability to prevent suffering such as Rob's downhill living hell.

However, just days after I learned of Rob's death, I read a new paper by Dr. Peter Nydahl, a respected PhD nurse in Europe, showing that in 116 ICUs across Germany, only 0.2 percent of ventilated patients were being walked despite clear evidence that early mobility helps speed patient recovery. The new way wasn't being adopted there at all. I felt a flash of anger. If that was true in a country as technologically and medically advanced as Germany, what hope was there for the rest of the world? Dr. Nydahl was devastated by what the study showed. And not just by the numbers on paper, but what his findings meant for all those patients whose lives would be impacted far into the future. "It was like standing in the dark, putting on a light, and seeing for the first time what is in the room," he told me. "We had so much work to do."

• • •

Since my first day of taking care of Sarah Bollich at Charity Hospital, I have been fascinated by the arc of critical illness. As a trainee and beyond, the pulse of my days was calibrated toward saving lives, and every action reflected this. When patients were rushed in with organs plummeting toward failure, we responded with rapid interventions, "lining and tubing them up," as we called it, and started them on life support.

If a patient deteriorated, we brought in more and more interventions: multiple lines and catheters, dialysis machines. When the patient was no longer in critical condition, we started to remove everything we had added. This might be days or weeks after the patient's ICU admission. Now that we had saved the patient's life, we would start to think about next steps.

That was the old way. Only later, when I began to understand the ramifications of all those interventions on my patients' lives, did I think of critical care as having a front and a back end. If the front end was the flurry of hands-on lifesaving care such as intubation and placing a central line, then the back end was the quality-of-life care such as early mobility. With the new way, we started to shift the back-end thinking to earlier in the arc. As soon as a patient entered the ICU, we knew we needed to consider more than keeping him alive. We wanted to have our eyes on long-term physical and mental health outcomes, too, and for me that meant that by the time the sun rose on the second ICU day, after the patient was stabilized, I was thinking about eliminating or lessening our front-end interventions. If it was safe and feasible—determined on a patient-by-patient basis—the team would remove or reduce chemical and physical restraints, immobilization, and isolation. The aim was to liberate the patient. As British medical ethicist Gordon Dunstan said, "The success of intensive care is not to be measured only by the statistics of survival, as though each death were a medical failure. It is to be measured by the quality of lives preserved or restored."

In practice, I knew it was hard to perfect this calibration. By 2014, however, we had started to make great strides. At Vanderbilt, we had redesigned our ICUs, a huge undertaking spearheaded by Dr. Art Wheeler, one of the directors of the medical ICU. They were spacious, practical, and filled with light. Each of the 150 upgraded rooms included a comfortable area for family members or friends to sit and sleep beside a patient's bed. The bathrooms were now large enough for a walk-in shower, ready for a patient to use, assisted, as soon as he was extubated. There were parquet floors, paintings on the walls, and beds that played music and spoke different languages. And I now knew that if a patient spoke the Lao language—or any other language—we had an interpreter on call for it. I had advocated for this myself. We invited family members to bring in personal items—photographs, blankets, books, and homemade posters—to make the rooms more familiar. It was all much friendlier for everyone, a long way from the sterile and alienating rooms the patients had suffered in before.

Dr. Art Wheeler and Dr. Todd Rice, the other director of our medical ICU, were proponents of bringing in early mobility. They were well respected by our entire critical care community, and their leadership set the tone for a fresh approach.

It was a thrill to watch our physical therapist, Elena Schiro, at work. It's not always simple to convince very sick patients to get out of bed, but she did it, easing their worries, cheering them on. I often saw her and a nurse walking with a patient to the end of the hall and back, a ventilator trailing behind, the sight that had cheered me so much in Odense. Elena worked in tandem with our occupational therapist, Brittany Work, whose role was to help with daily living skills. She would spend time talking to patients, playing tic-tac-toe or hangman with them, engaging their brains. Sometimes I would hear her in conversation: "So, Mr. Lancaster, you tell me you like fishing. . . . Trout fishing. Can you write a list of the things you would need for your next trip? . . . Bait, yes. . . . Night crawlers, okay, then." Mr. Lancaster was writing in his notebook, his face serious as he concentrated on the words, then his eyes on her face while she looked over his list. "Coffee, that's a good one," Brittany said with a laugh. It looked nonmedical, yet I knew the good it was doing her patient's brain. Actively rebuilding connections between neurons that had been severed during his illness. And mending his spirit. I hoped he was thinking beyond his ICU bed to those early-morning fishing trips he might enjoy soon enough, the mist rising off the river. Seeing the joy both Brittany and Elena experienced through their work, I imagined it was good for them, too. They were staunch patient advocates and had recently attended critical care rehabilitation conferences to increase their knowledge. It felt like progress. It also felt like a beginning. I wondered if we were to conduct a study across the United States, as Peter Nydahl had across Germany, what percentage of the nation's critical care patients were being treated the new way. What if we were to turn on the lights?

• • •

On December 9, 1999, Dr. Donald Berwick, the founder, president, and CEO of the Institute for Healthcare Improvement (IHI), delivered a memorable speech at the 11th Annual National Forum on Quality Improvement (QI) in Health Care. In his address, he told the story of the 1949 Mann Gulch wildfire in Montana, which took the lives of thirteen young firefighters, then applied the lessons learned from that tragedy to health care. Berwick's wife, Ann, was treated in the hospital for a serious condition that year, and he had realized the many ways in which the health-care system needed to change, as I had when my daughter was hospitalized. The first time I read his speech was over twelve years later when I was working with Kelly McCutcheon Adams, a trauma ICU social worker and a director at the IHI. Kelly was building a team for a quality-improvement series called "Rethinking Critical Care: Decreasing Sedation, Increasing Delirium Monitoring, and Increasing Patient Mobility," and I was excited to accept her invitation to jump aboard. We were trying to expand the new approach to critical care to different ICUs by conducting multiple hands-on teaching seminars across the country.

I had been riveted by *Young Men and Fire*, Norman Maclean's account of the Mann Gulch tragedy. Fifteen smoke jumpers and one fireguard took on what appeared to be a containable fire that instead grew into a forty-five-hundred-acre blaze. After the men parachuted in, the wind changed direction and the flames burst toward them. Against the odds, they all made a run for it, except for team leader Wagner "Wag" Dodge, who did something so radical that it seemed like complete idiocy: he used a match to light a new fire in the grass right in front of the main fire. As soon as the grass burned, Dodge lay facedown while the howling flames raced around him, lifting him feetfirst into the air, then slamming him safely and untouched into the fresh ashes. While Dodge had yelled for others to follow him into his escape fire, no one had listened. Only Dodge and two members of his team survived.

Many errors were made that day in Mann Gulch, and as I read through Berwick's speech, I felt inspired by his wisdom. He believed five preconditions were required to achieve a successful culture of safety in medicine: facing reality, dropping old tools, staying in formation, communicating better, and developing capable leadership. He asked, "Now we have a chance. What does the escape fire look like?"

As Kelly and I moved forward with our workshops, these ideas were at the forefront of my mind. I had accepted the reality that the old ways of treating our patients in the ICU had engulfed patients either in the hospital or in their lives after discharge. Now we were poised to use new tools to help ICUs adopt a culture of safety. I was pleased to work with the IHI, whose mission is one of quality improvement for health and health care worldwide. In essence, this means bridging the chasm between the care we *are* getting, and the care we *should be* getting.

It felt good to be following in the footsteps of Dr. Avedis Donabedian, the father of quality assessment in health care, to try to find the most effective ways for hospitals to deliver the best care to patients and to make the greatest positive difference in their lives. At each workshop we brought attendees—doctors, nurses, physical therapists, respiratory therapists, everyone who works with critically ill patients—right into the action of ICU rooms to learn from real patients. With the scientific data and papers already out in medical journals, we wanted to demonstrate how the changes impacted patients in their lives. I wanted people to be captivated by the humanity of what they saw.

Hundreds of medical centers had signed on to change their standard practices by following a multistep protocol called the ABCDEs of Critical Care, built upon the foundation of our own ABC *Lancet* study and other papers. In the spirit of Malcolm Gladwell's *The Tipping Point*, we wanted the set of practices to be "sticky" to the brain, easy to remember together. We had assigned the first five letters of the alphabet: *A* reminded ICU teams to assess analgesia (presence of pain), to prevent and manage each patient's pain; *B* addressed both spontaneous awakening and spontaneous breathing trials (stopping sedation and then stopping the ventilator each morning); *C* referred to the choice of pain and sedation medications, trying when possible to avoid drugs such as benzodiazepines that lead to so much delirium; *D* ensured that teams would assess, prevent, and manage delirium; and *E* stood for early mobility and exercise (getting patients out of bed as soon as possible in the ICU stay). Later we would use the term *bundle* for the protocol, once we had proved that the different elements saved lives and reduced harm when performed collectively and reliably.

We started out with just thirty attendees in 2011 in Salt Lake City. Kelly's team consisted of Polly Bailey and Dr. Terry Clemmer, and we had added Vicki Spuhler, a senior critical care nurse manager from Intermountain, and a fiery, veteran physical therapist from the University of California, San Francisco, named Heidi Engel. They could rouse even the greatest doubters and provide a spark of hope when the walls of resistance seemed too high. As we traveled to Washington, DC, San Diego, Chicago, and San Francisco with our seminars, it began to feel like a mission. Changing minds and saving lives, one patient at a time. Or one doctor, who saw new possibilities in practice and took that promise home to her own ICU team. One nurse inspired by what he saw, a physical therapist determined to share what she had learned. I imagined ripples of hope washing from hospital to hospital. I wanted everyone who came to the workshops to feel the same excitement I'd experienced in Odense.

It was ingrained in my mind to write up the science so that others could learn, so I sought out several hospitals that were eager to both change their ICU culture and document and report their results. We followed their progress. The team from Samaritan Hospital in Troy, New York, described its ICU care before attending the conferences: "All our ventilated patients received continuous infusions of narcotics and benzodiazepines to the point that there was no limb movement, no awakening assessments, and no regard for delirium whatsoever." At that time, this description could have applied to most critical care units across the country. As the different ICU teams tried to follow the new protocols, they recorded their successes and challenges as they explored the difficulties of real-world application of evidence-based practices at the bedside. We knew there would be struggles: changing cultures and human practices was never easy. Their hurdles were predictable. Some team members were often reluctant to acknowledge that their current standard care was not the best way. "I've been doing critical care for twenty years!" said one senior nurse. "What's wrong with my approach?" Some genuinely feared that turning off sedation earlier would terrify patients, or cause them to pull out their tubes, or make them dangerous to staff, or that walking ventilated patients would hurt them. The idea that a patient's quality of life might be affected after discharge seemed too far away to focus on, too invisible to worry about. Coordinating interdisciplinary teams to provide care caused struggles as well. And it seemed like a huge amount of work.

In response, we acknowledged that change was difficult. We also taught people how to set themselves up for success, and to start with easy wins. To choose the frequently admitted emphysema patient without wounds or broken limbs, or an uncomplicated postoperative patient, when starting to mobilize, rather than the multisystem-trauma patient with a broken pelvis. To understand that one negative experience was just that; following protocols could and should still continue. To find champions among staff members, those who would cheer on the team. To take a deep breath and quietly remind ourselves that doing something one way for so long doesn't make it right. Mostly, we observed that when teams saw the transformative power of waking up patients and walking them on the ventilator, they said they would never go back to the old ways.

The mobility part was often the hardest element to implement, and when it happened, it felt celebratory; it was usually the result of extraordinary effort and teamwork. The staff at Rapid City Regional Hospital in South Dakota told us the story of one of their sickest patients, a critically ill, intubated woman on dialysis around the clock for acute kidney injury. "By her third day, the mobility team had her standing, out of bed, and marching in place right next to her dialysis machine. This was something we thought we would never see, but we did it!" Their sense of achievement was palpable.

One of the mantras at the IHI was "What can you do by next Tuesday?" It was especially helpful in countering feelings of being overwhelmed by the idea of implementing so much change. We followed the Plan-Do-Study-Act (PDSA) cycles model. On Mondays the teams would gather and plan a small change, implement it on Tuesday, then study what worked and what didn't. We would continue with changes that showed improvements, while acknowledging the benefits of knowing what didn't. I had always been a person who wanted everything to happen quickly, to bring on all the change at one time. It was good to be taught by Kelly that small tests of change were much more effective and sustainable.

Against seemingly insurmountable odds set up by decades of errant thought, seeing individual patients' lives turned around and hearing heartfelt testimonies from staff and families made believers of dozens of health-care workers across the country. With Dr. Berwick and the rest of the Boston-based IHI troupe whispering in her ear, Kelly McCutcheon Adams lit an escape fire.

• • •

"It's not enough to keep people from dying. We have to save the life that they want to return to, the one they had before they came to us." This was critical care nurse Mary Ann Barnes-Daly's mantra when she led a multicenter study across the Sutter Health hospital system, headquartered in Sacramento, California. Seven community hospitals had received a grant from the Gordon and Betty Moore Foundation to study the association between ABCDEF bundle compliance and patient outcomes. Family engagement and empowerment (*F*) was a new addition to the bundle and was crucially important. Gordon Moore, cofounder of Intel Corporation, had spent some time suffering with delirium in the ICU not too long before and had found the absence of his family hugely distressing. He wanted to be sure that others would have open access to their families as a healing presence and insisted that we increase bedside contact with loved ones. I was more than happy to include family involvement as a cornerstone of the bundle, and we decided to invite family members to daily rounds with the ICU teams, in addition to implementing open visitation. I could see that this engagement should have been there all along. It was another important step in letting my gaze move beyond the organ and the body to the patients, and then further outward to see their family.

I first met Mary Ann the same day I heard Debra and Anthony Russo tell their story of his decline after his ICU stay. They were a powerful reminder that we needed to succeed in getting the bundle implemented: no matter what the science behind the new way showed, it was only useful if it reached our patients. To her friends, Mary Ann was known as Jett, and her no-nonsense, scrappy honesty seemed to fit with this. The ICU teams would have no chance of noncompliance with her in charge. In 2014, under her leadership, the Sutter Health hospital teams enrolled 6,064 patients and undertook the first multicenter study of the ABCDEFs of critical care, which was built using over thirty-five individual studies from the *New England Journal of Medicine*, *JAMA*, and the *Lancet*. When all was said and done, the Sutter Health project was the first to show that higher compliance with the ABCDEF approach, which we came to call the A2F bundle, yielded higher survival rates and more time free of coma and delirium.

Jett told me how she had approached changing the culture of critical care within her hospital system. "I went to the ICU in my small hospital and told them about the bundle. 'Here's A and B and C,' and I explained everything, and the nurses nodded: 'Uh-huh, uh-huh.' I said, 'So this is what we have to do. This is the new cool stuff.' They said, 'Great.' Two weeks later I went back, and you know what they had done? Nothing." Jett laughed. I could imagine she didn't laugh at the time, though. "Trying to sell people on mortality reduction isn't really meaningful to them. You have to sell patients' stories." That was exactly what we had learned, too. You must sell stories to get people on board.

Jett went on, "I went to our flagship hospital, Sutter Medical Center, where there was an ICU nursing meet. There had to be sixty or seventy nurses in the room. I had an hour. I spent forty minutes talking to them about how we were hurting patients, and twenty minutes on how we're going to fix it. I told them what sedation did. I told them what tying patients down in bed did, how they couldn't walk or have their jobs or how they lost their spouses and their families. How they said they'd rather be dead. I had nurses crying. They'd thought they were doing the right thing because that's what we'd been taught. They said, 'We didn't know.' I said, 'I didn't know. I'm learning all this stuff, too. But we're hurting people, we're breaking their brains.'"

Jett had tears in her eyes as she remembered. She looked back at me. "That's what got people hooked."

Now I can't imagine the bundle without family engagement and empowerment, and I wonder why it took so long to realize that not all healing comes from the medical team. It had struck me time and time again how we were losing the patients' voices in their own narratives, but I hadn't made the leap to understand how families could help their loved ones—and in doing so could help their ICU teams. I saw families work with nurses and physical and occupational therapists to reorient patients when they awoke from sedation, cheer patients on as they made the move from hospital bed to chair, play word games with them and read to them from their favorite books or magazines to keep their brains engaged. I realized that families had knowledge about their loved ones that we could never have known, and that it was important to their healing. They were a crucial part of the team.

The Moore Foundation went on to fund the ICU Liberation Collaborative of the Society of Critical Care Medicine (SCCM), which took ownership of the A2F safety bundle. The collaborative—so called because patients were being liberated not just from the ventilator but also from delirium, chemical and physical restraints, their bed, and the entire negative ICU experience—enrolled 15,226 patients in 68 adult and 10 pediatric ICUs across the United States and Puerto Rico from 2015 to early 2017. For those two years, we introduced the A2F bundle to them, following the same steps of changing the culture I'd learned from the IHI by building teams, finding champions, conducting small tests of change, monitoring compliance, and winning local buy-in through seeing work in action. Over fifteen thousand patients received the new way of care, which impacted not only their lives and their loved ones', but also their health-care teams' lives.

One of the original nurse leaders of the bundle, Dr. Michele Balas, as well as Dr. Brenda Pun, Chris Perme, and Heidi Engel, spent hours in hospitals across the country with the teams and families, fanning the flame of their local escape fires. Their stories were heartwarming. One father of a young woman on life support played videos on his iPad of Muppet, their dog, his happy bark rising above the ding of machines. How he laughed and cried when his daughter came out of sedation and the first thing she wrote on her whiteboard was "Muppet?" A firefighter in the ICU with his brother who had suffered a heart attack was grateful to know that rounds were at 9:00 a.m. every day, that he could be there and be included as part of the team, before heading into work.

In the old way, ICUs limited family members' access to loved ones, and we shared only the knowledge we thought necessary or that we felt we had the time to give. Now we understand that this was a kind of testimonial injustice; we had devalued the family and taken away their right to have a say in a loved one's care by consolidating power solely within the confines of the medical team. With ICU Liberation and the A2F bundle, we not only expanded but leveraged the value in having family—and patients—as core members of each ICU team.

Our own Nashville Veterans Affairs hospital was one of two VA medical centers in the ICU Liberation Collaborative, and nurse leader Kelly Drumright was quick to embrace and champion the bundle. She liked the humanism at its core. She saw the way it ultimately brings about patient autonomy, enabling the patient to voice unmet physical, emotional, and spiritual needs. She especially welcomed the opportunity for family to be at their loved ones' bedsides, having gone through a distressing experience during her own father's death a few years earlier. She and other family members were denied full access to him while he was dying.

I watched her fight to change the old culture, working with nurses who were steeped in the old ways. Some were combative, and some left their jobs. But she persevered. She found that sharing videos—with permission—of the patients' progress made a huge difference in motivating her team. Seeing Mr. Wood sedated on day one and being scooted into his bedside chair with help from his physical therapist on day three resonated. The nurses could see that their hard work was paying off. Physician leader Dr. Julie Bastarache played an important part, too, assigning a doctor to oversee each letter of the bundle and even purchasing a wheeled device to carry the ventilated patients' medical equipment as each of them made daily laps around our rectangular ICU.

• • •

One of the most convincing things in all of medicine is when we see both a dose response and the same answer across multiple studies. A dose response simply means that a higher dose of something, such as a medication, works better than a lower dose (or vice versa). One can also deliver different "doses" of a clinical intervention by being more or less compliant with a protocol. Just as in the Sutter experience, the SCCM's ICU Liberation Collaborative showed that the more the entire A2F bundle was employed, the less time patients spent in the ICU and hospital, the more often they lived, and the more time they spent free of coma and delirium. For the twenty-one thousand patients in the two studies, the six treatment steps also meant more time mobilizing out of bed, fewer ICU readmissions, fewer nursing home transfers, and more discharges to home, where patients could return to the life they had before they came to us. Just as Jett and all of us had wanted.

When I started my research into delirium, I was concerned primarily with discovering the potential causes of this brain injury, and things I might be doing to make it worse. Ultimately, I hoped to prevent it, or at least mitigate its effects. I underestimated how helpful my journey in developing the A2F bundle would be in finding my way back to my patients. In 2018, our National Institute on Aging–sponsored MIND-USA study, published in the *New England Journal of Medicine*, showed for the first time that antipsychotics such as haloperidol—the most used treatment for delirium in hospitals and nursing homes for the past forty years—did not lessen delirium in critically ill patients. These results were especially important to our desire to bring patient-centered care to ICUs across the world. No longer would doctors and ICU teams believe they were doing enough for their patients' delirium by writing a prescription for a drug. Now they were forced to reckon with the data that the best reduction of delirium in the ICU is from the six steps of the A2F bundle: control pain, lessen sedation, wake people up, manage delirium, mobilize early, and involve family. Follow the science and find the humanity. The bundle had helped me to see the person in the patient, the human inside the hospital gown.

As the person-centered care at the core of the bundle became more widely used across the United States, I traveled to multiple countries around the world to speak with and support doctors and hospital leaders who were ready to embrace change. They had read our papers with interest and were eager to implement elements of the bundle into their own patient care. It was thrilling to behold. When we conducted a survey, led by Stradivarius-loving geriatrician Dr. Alessandro Morandi, of 1,521 ICUs in 47 countries on 6 continents, it showed that parts of the bundle had been incorporated into bedside practice by as many as 89 percent of the ICUs, while only 57 percent had implemented the entire A2F safety package. Although the survey had shone a light on the magnitude of the effort that still lay ahead, I was excited to see that our work was beginning to spread across the United States and around the globe.

A colleague of mine, Dr. Raul Alejandro Gomez, an insightful physician and thought leader in Latin America, once came up to me at a conference in Buenos Aires and said, "It seems to me the 'classic' care of critically ill patients is similar to a dementia factory. It is up to us to close this factory." We were on our way.

• • •

A couple of years ago on rounds, I met a new patient with a skin infection in the corner of her left eye.

"Good morning, Mrs. Keith, I'm Dr. Ely and we are going to take care of you."

Bill and Janet Keith had dated through high school and college and, now in their seventies, had been married for over fifty years. They held hands. I could see they were scared. When the infection had spread quickly from her left ear to her eye, she was rushed by ambulance and admitted to our ICU. Over the next few hours, as the infection raged like wildfire across her face, it became clear to our team that she had necrotizing fasciitis. The same disease that had started on Rob Harmer's elbow. Surgeons raced to remove the dying skin on her face down to the muscle layers, trying to keep a step ahead of the disease. One surgery led to two, then more, until most of the skin was gone. Then, in much the same way as Rob's, her body was overwhelmed by septic shock, ARDS, and kidney failure, and we hurried to put her on life support, her room filling with machines and tubes. Her cheeks and eye sockets were riddled with tiny two-millimeter drainage tubes, a breathing tube in her throat connected her to the ventilator, and a panel of IV pumps sent no less than fifteen medications into her body to keep her alive.

Next to Janet's bed were photographs in frames. Of her and Bill and their grown-up sons, Bo and Mike, with their families. There she was, surrounded by her grandchildren. In one photograph, she was dressed in a long gown and sparkling jewelry. In another, I noticed the Eiffel Tower. "We love to travel," said Bill in his thick Southern drawl. "Every occasion we get." He was a constant presence in the room, settled into the family area or sitting by Janet's bed, talking softly to her. "We have a lot to talk about," he said. I urged, "Keep going. She can hear you." Often the sons were there, support for Janet, for Bill, for each other, taking turns sitting at the bedside.

I began whispering in her ear, "Janet, I'm taking care of all of you. Your mind, body, and spirit." I couldn't tell if she registered my words, but I continued, "You are a woman of grace, and in order to get you out of here and back to your life, you need to be a refined badass." I wasn't sure why I said it, but Bill had told me she had a sense of humor. As soon as she was stable enough, we sat her up in bed and then started her walking. She fought against us, but with Bill rooting for her and with help from her nurses and physical therapist, we walked her all the way down the hall, the ventilator following behind. Her huge bandage across her eyes and face earned her the nickname Lone Ranger from the staff, and they would coax her forward. Bill was always there, saying, "Honey, I love you and am right here with you. The boys are here, too, and the grandkids are at home waiting for you to hug them again." Often her delirium was so dense that she gave no response other than a brief nod. But he kept going, always encouraging, and so did we, with our focus on treating the many elements of her critical illness, guided by the A2F bundle, making sure we protected her brain and her body, too. We used light sedation when she needed it, and then, as soon as she passed her spontaneous breathing trial, we extubated her and liberated her from the ventilator. That meant she could have a shower, something so basic and yet quintessentially uplifting. Janet's first words to me were "Dr. Ely, I never stopped hearing your words, and they drove me to become that 'refined badass' you wanted me to be. It saved my life."

The most striking thing I learned as a physician over the years had nothing to do with science or data. It was one patient story at a time. With the evolution of our work, I reread Avedis Donabedian's work on quality improvement. I was certain he'd distill the best way forward, and he did not disappoint: "Systems awareness and systems design are important for health professionals but are not enough. They are enabling mechanisms only. It is the ethical dimension of individuals that is essential to a system's success. Ultimately, the secret of quality is love."

Chapter 11

Finding the Person in the Patient—Hope through Humanization

> *Compassion was the most important, perhaps the sole law of human existence.*

> —Fyodor Dostoyevsky, *The Idiot*

FOR THE PAST EIGHT years, I have enjoyed an early-morning ritual, when I can, of biking in our neighborhood with Butter, our new dog. A yellow Lab mix rescue, named after our love of rich New Orleans desserts, I hold her leash in my left hand and steer the handlebars with my right. A neighbor tried this and ended up with a broken wrist, but I think I have it down. Butter bounds beside me, her tongue sliding sideways out of her grin. On the ride, I try to keep my thoughts outward, taking in the stars as they fade toward morning or watching the arrival of a blue-skied day.

When Butter and I return home, I keep the workday at bay for a little longer, taking time for meditation, then sitting with Kim before we head to the hospital. After rounding on my patients, I change focus, often dictating emails, texts, and notes to myself, and others. When I read them through later, I notice that the initialism *ICU* often appears as "I see you." At first, I cringed whenever this error showed up, turning my careful prose into gibberish. I felt the need to send follow-up emails and apologies. But now I just smile. It's always good to be reminded of our primary goal in critical care: to make our patients feel seen, their voices heard.

My friend Dr. Gabriel Heras La Calle, a well-known intensivist in Madrid, Spain, and founder/director of the Humanizing Intensive Care project (Proyecto HU-CI), describes the intensive care unit as a depersonalization chamber: a place in which people are stripped of their individuality, their life story, their needs and values. In short, everything that makes them who they are is grayed out. Recently Dr. Heras shared a striking graphic with me—created, we believe, by Dr. Thomas Morrow—of people speeding on a conveyor belt into a chamber, where they are transformed into generic gowned patients before emerging, ready to be received by their health-care teams. Their aspirations and idiosyncrasies, preferences and memories, have disappeared. Each day I try not to let that happen. I like to keep in mind a phrase Dr. Heras taught me: *"Cada persona es un mundo."* "Each person is a world." I have come a long way since I viewed my patient as a lung to be fixed, and I find it almost unbelievable now to look back at that "other me" with a laser-beam focus on a patient's collapsing organs. With scientific precision, I used to home in on the problem, seeing my patient through the lens of her CT scan or her X-ray, reduced to a purely physical depiction of self. I thought I was cutting through the noise. Now I know the noise matters, too.

As a medical student, I was taught to take a social history of my patients just after the history of present illness and past medical history. This was the moment when, in theory, we would learn the backstories that personalize our patients. In reality, doctors are busy, and the social history ended up minimized to a few questions: How far did you go in school and what is your profession? What diseases run in your family? Do you smoke, drink, or do drugs? The questions were not intended as conversation starters, and in many cases, given the intensity of critical illness and the overhanging shadow of death, they were never asked at all.

Now with my patients awake and alert earlier in their stay and less likely to be delirious, the atmosphere has changed in the ICU. We doctors are still busy, and we still feel the need to move on to the next intervention, but our patients are often present and looking at us, so conversations can occur. I see nurses bantering as they find out whom they are caring for, asking family for information to deepen the interactions—something they do now even before our patients are awake. I was bothered that doctors and nurses on television shows were way ahead of us on this. For years, writers had given patients carefully scripted backstories, messy love lives and complicated family dynamics, the things that make us root for them and for the doctors to save them.

As I've grown older, I have allowed myself to move from a purely cerebral approach at the bedside to a more emotional one. I've come to understand that my medical knowledge and technical skills are important in caring for my patients, but alone they are not good enough. Now I want to open myself up to what my patient is feeling and thinking, and to how I can best support his needs.

Dr. Heras told me he once heard a Spanish celebrity complain, after a prolonged hospital stay, that the ICU is a "branch of hell." Shocked that someone would say this after having his life saved, Dr. Heras was motivated to find out more. He surveyed ICU survivors, doctors, and nurses and studied their answers. We call this qualitative research because we're studying quality and the narrative of people's thoughts and beliefs, instead of measuring numbers and rates—which is quantitative research. Some consider qualitative research warm and fuzzy, but when done well, it is vitally important. The celebrity's negative reaction to his hospital stay was not unusual among ICU patients. What's more, Dr. Heras and his colleagues realized that if doctors and nurses were lying in ICU beds, they, too, would feel fear, pain, loneliness, confusion, and loss of dignity and identity. Patients, regardless of their backgrounds, were thirsty, too hot or too cold, exhausted, and unable to communicate. These were not complicated issues to resolve, but they did require a different mind-set, one that became the cornerstone of Dr. Heras's Humanizing Intensive Care.

As a global critical care community, we came to understand that ICU care is not all rush and noise and life-or-death intensity. We needed to slow down, take the time to smile at a patient, hold her hand, and acknowledge that she was scared. To listen and readjust a pillow. To take a moment to open the blinds in the morning to let the spring day stream in. I think of this as our "bigger fish to fry" error in judgment. We thought we could consider personalized care optional or expendable, a mind-set I was taught and then came to model, indicating, "I don't have time for that! I'm saving lives here!" And there was some justification in thinking that way. Every day in the ICU, we're juggling so much—patients going into shock or needing to be reintubated—and our medical interventions in those instances seem more vital. But we are not always in crisis mode, and we must take the time to provide this equally important person-centered care. To understand what matters to each patient. What's more, we now understand that keeping the whole person in our vision helps to mitigate our patients' delirium and improves their medical outcomes.

Another way we've taken personal needs into account is to alter medication schedules or forgo nighttime baths (it's now hard for me to imagine that we used to schedule baths at 3:00 a.m. because the team had more time then) so a patient can sleep. Disrupted sleep in the ICU is believed to contribute to delirium. Studies show that many ICU patients get less than one hour of good sleep per day due to constant interruptions for tests, noise from many sources including alarms, machines, and staff conversations, outside lights, and side effects from medications. Sedatives, including benzodiazepines and propofol, cause slow-wave-sleep suppression, reducing anabolic—restorative—rapid eye movement (REM) sleep. The absence of this slow-wave sleep can further injure patients.

With an explosion of research, we have come to realize how vitally important sleep is to health. Just as our body cleans our blood using the lymphatic system, the brain clears out toxins through the glymphatic system. While we are still learning about glymphatic fluid movements, early work suggests that it may not activate fully in the human brain until specific stages of the sleep cycle. Thus, short sleep times may reduce the effectiveness of our brain's "waste disposal" pathway. There is some evidence that sedation and anesthesia impair glymphatic flow as well. In the ICU, this could put a patient's already injured brain at greater risk of acquiring dementia or send a patient closer to death.

ICU sleep protocols or "nap times" are being devised and studied by Drs. Melissa Knauert and Margaret Pisani at Yale School of Medicine. By understanding sources of disruption and prioritizing sleep for at least four hours from midnight to 4:00 a.m., they were able to reduce noise by one-third and significantly lessen interruptions. However, they noted that for some extremely ill patients, four hours of uninterrupted sleep was just not feasible. While sleep protocols often conflict with ICU culture and practice on many levels, we will have to be mindful and work harder to integrate them into our current care systems.

We are also learning to introduce the healing energy of music into our ICUs, harnessing its power to reduce anxiety and fear in our patients. Music also distracts them from the general noise and stress of an ICU stay, while often evoking happy memories, far beyond their current situation. It's simple to provide headphones for patients or to stream music in their rooms on various devices and allow them, or their loved ones, to choose their own playlist. I have found that it provides an easy entry point to forming a connection. One patient wanted to listen to the soundtrack from his favorite movie trilogy, *The Lord of the Rings*, and I remember the blissful smile that spread across his face as the first bars of "The Shire" echoed through his room. Later, after extubation, I found him in conversation with one of our nurses discussing their favorite scenes.

ICU diaries are another way to facilitate personal connections. Think of how much we learned from Anne Frank's remarkable diary.

Her detailed memories of her family's torturous experience of their time in hiding offer a unique perspective on a dark period in history. Dr. Carl Bäckman, a Swedish PhD nurse, first published an intriguing idea in 2001 that is like a mirror image of *The Diary of Anne Frank*. If a person experiencing harrowing events was unable to write them down, others could keep a journal to help her put the puzzle pieces together later. This is the concept of an ICU diary, created by a critically ill patient's loved ones and medical team and including words, pictures, sometimes even videos of events that occur during an ICU stay. PhD nurse/scientist Dr. Christina Jones, a pioneer in critical care, partnered with Dr. Bäckman to publish the first randomized trial in 2010 testing this concept. The diaries worked to reduce the development of PTSD in critical care survivors from 13 percent in the control group down to 5 percent in those who received these detailed notes on their hospital stays.

ICU diaries give family members an important activity and purpose during long hours at a loved one's bedside and help patients process their hospital stay after discharge. What I hadn't realized was how they would help me as a doctor. The handwritten notes remind me that my patients have a life beyond their ICU room, filled with moments and people that are important to them. Recently, a diary entry caught my eye. Written by an old friend of my patient, it thanked her for the time she scored their team's winning run in a high school state championship softball game. The friend continued that this victory had given her the confidence at a critical time to do more with her life. When my patient awoke from a nap, I asked about the big game. She perked up in a way I hadn't seen before, and suddenly I had access into her world.

When I write my own diary entries or personal notes to my patients, I know they are not a part of the medical record, so I am able to express my thoughts freely. A recent diary entry I wrote said, "Tisha, just a reminder for when you wake up: that fear you were having about someone coming to hurt you is not real. You are loved, and we are here to care for you as you get better and come off this ventilator. I'll see you later today." I asked the nurse to please show it to Tisha as soon as she woke up in the hopes we might alleviate her anxiety.

When I was a young doctor, I would have dismissed the idea that sleep, music, or diary writing might be part of my tool kit as an intensivist, one that I would readily use to benefit my patients. Now I know better. Our patients are people and respond to person-centered care.

For decades, John Prine has been one of my favorite singer-songwriters, and when he went down with COVID-19, it was an honor for Vanderbilt's ICU team to look after him. Revered and beloved by many millions worldwide, he didn't ask for any special treatment, not even when his illness took a turn for the worse, which didn't surprise us. He was true to whom he had been all his life. We cared for him as we cared for all our patients, trying our best to save him, knowing how precious he was to his loved ones. When it became clear that his prognosis was dire, that his double pneumonia would overwhelm his body, and that he would die, his team focused on making him feel safe until the end. He passed away on April 7, 2020. A few months after his death, I spoke with Fiona Whelan Prine, his widow—they were married for twenty-three years—about the life and love they shared. Many years earlier, John had turned down an appearance on the Larry King show because, as Fiona told me, "he had no intention of ever becoming a person who couldn't wear his dirty black T-shirt to Kroger's." She laughed at the memory. I imagined that if John had gone through a depersonalization chamber before his admission to the ICU, he would have been reduced to "celebrity" or "musician." Which he was, and there was no escaping it. Instead, we were able to see his humanity, his hopes, fears and needs; his boundless love for Fiona, conveyed once more in the last song he wrote, "I Remember Everything." She told me the nurses treated John as though he were their father, and she was grateful. She added, "Because of the difficulty of dealing with a disease without a vaccine, or therapeutics at the time, with no cure, certainly, all that's left is heart. All there is, is humanity. All there is, is caring."

• • •

Titus Lansing was just four years old when he developed flu symptoms that led to his whole body shutting down within days, and an emergency helicopter ride to Children's Hospital at Vanderbilt. Doctors and nurses there told his parents, Alison and Matt, that Titus wouldn't likely make it through the night. He was immediately intubated, then an ECMO machine was added, taking his blood outside his body to add oxygen and remove carbon dioxide before reintroducing it into his veins. When his kidneys failed, his doctors started continuous dialysis. When he went into cardiac arrest, an emergency team rushed in to resuscitate his small body, which was overwhelmed by septic shock. He barely survived the code blue, and Matt and Alison prepared for the worst. They hadn't thought about what to tell Titus's siblings: his twin sister, Caroline, and his six-year-old brother, Wylie. Everything happened too fast.

Astonishingly, Titus pulled through. His recovery took six weeks in the pediatric ICU and another three weeks of rehab in Atlanta. His physician, pediatric intensivist Dr. Kristina Betters, told me the team was scared Titus would lose his ability to walk if they didn't get him out of bed and moving. Fortunately, Dr. Betters was part of the Pediatric ICU Liberation team at Vanderbilt, led by Dr. Heidi Smith, a fierce advocate of the A2F bundle, who adapted and validated a pediatric version of our delirium tool. "Titus was an early mobility superstar!" Dr. Betters said. They brought in physical therapists, occupational therapists, and a speech therapist to work on communication. His parents were constantly at his bedside. Dr. Betters helped sit Titus in a tiny chair at a low table, with Caroline and Wylie on a play mat on the floor, so they could all build LEGOs together. "That was the first time they interacted with each other," said Alison. "Before that they were terrified." It was an extraordinarily difficult experience for their family.

When the family arrived home in Madison, Alabama, a town of

just forty-five thousand people, Titus was a local celebrity. Everywhere they went, people called him the miracle boy. He was the boy who lived. But for Alison and her family, the only familiar thing about life was their dog, Chewy, named after Chewbacca from *Star Wars*. Matt designs rockets for NASA, and it felt as if the whole family had ended up on a distant planet. When Titus was in the ICU, Alison's friends had given her a box of goodies with chocolate and some little bottles of liquor. "I don't even drink, but we got home that first night, and Titus was screaming because we were trying to change his dressings. Caroline was screaming because Titus was getting attention, and Wylie was screaming and crying about I don't know what. Well, I ran into my office and dug through that box to get the liquor out."

Even with the best treatment in the ICU, recovery is still difficult. Post-ICU interventions are a crucial part of an ongoing care plan. It's been a year now since Titus went home. He is back in school, back to being a kid who loves trying out Jedi moves with his new light saber. But the ordeal of his hospital stay is far from behind him or the rest of the family. Titus still struggles with ongoing weakness and pain in his feet, legs, and arms. He has nightmares about bandage changes and blood draws. He panics if rough play nearby might hurt him in some way. His sister, Caroline, worries about him constantly, always needing to know where he is, and has developed a chronic phantom foot pain of her own. Wylie has become protective of his little brother and is concerned about his parents dying. Both Alison and Matt have been diagnosed with PTSD, and the stress has caused Alison's Crohn's disease to flare up, leading to multiple hospitalizations in short order, adding to the children's anxiety. As Alison puts it, "There's just a whole lot of layers to our onion."

The Lansings' story feels familiar to me in many ways: critical illness barreling into someone's life and leaving devastation in its wake. Yet it is not this sense of déjà vu that strikes me. Instead it is the little things. The frozen pork chops that Alison can't bring herself to cook because they remind her of the night that Titus was taken to the hospital. That he was named after a preacher at their church in Cape Canaveral. That Caroline and Titus are twins, which especially resonates for me as I am the father of twins. That Matt is an actual rocket scientist. These are the things that make them who they are, the stories they carry with them, that make them human. This is what I am drawn to now as a doctor. Just as patients must receive personalized treatment in the ICU, their treatment on returning home must be personalized, too.

The Lansing family has PICS-F, a post-intensive care syndrome that affects family members of critical care patients. Dr. Betters anticipated this. As part of her care of Titus, she arranged for follow-up for him and his family at the CIBS Center—two hours away by car—so she and the team could oversee his post-ICU physical, cognitive, and mental health recovery. He receives physical therapy and psychological counseling, and the other members of the family are also undergoing individual therapy to help them process Titus's illness and the way it has impacted their lives. Sometimes family members feel guilty about struggling, as they weren't the ones who went through the ordeal of critical illness. Their pain must be validated, too. We have finally understood that the arc of critical illness reaches far into our patients' lives, beyond their hospital stays, and that it needs to be standard practice to provide care for them—and their families—down the line in a proactive way. We can't wait for them to struggle and then find their way back to us.

• • •

Dr. Carla Sevin, an intensivist at Vanderbilt, and a humanist at heart, was concerned about the impact PICS has in patients' lives and worked hard to launch the ICU Recovery Center, now widely known and part of our CIBS Center. Dr. Sevin skillfully steered our hospital administration toward granting space for the fledging clinic on Fridays when no one else wanted the rooms. One patient at a time, she and her interprofessional team began seeing survivors from our ICUs, starting with those who were at high risk for developing PICS. Patients who had been on a ventilator, in shock, or delirious were invited to her clinic for transitional care after discharge before being handed over—with records and recommendations—to their primary care physicians. It was a brilliant way to begin serving patients during the downstream portion of their critical illness. Many other leading hospitals around the country and world also opened similar post-ICU clinics to address the growing need, and this entire movement has been invigorated by the Society of Critical Care Medicine's THRIVE Initiative, led by visionaries such as Dr. Sevin, Dr. Jack Iwashyna at the University of Michigan in Ann Arbor, and Dr. Aluko Hope at the Albert Einstein College of Medicine in New York.

I am reminded again of my time years ago working with transplant patients. We understood that our patients would be replacing one set of problems—from a failing organ—with another set of problems after their surgery—from ongoing treatment to prevent organ rejection. We explained this to them and prepared a supportive clinical plan for post-surgery care. While critical illness usually sweeps in out of the blue, leaving little time for preparations, we already know that our patients will likely need long-term care and can quickly coordinate with an ICU recovery team.

Several specialties make up an ICU recovery center clinic, and ours includes an ICU doctor, pharmacy specialist, nurse practitioner, and psychologist. They work together to arrange physical and occupational therapy, reconcile long medication lists, tend to wound healing, address ongoing cognitive and mental health problems, make referrals to local doctors and specialists, and help with practical aspects of life such as insurance, employment, financial issues, and disability claims. Often our survivors are turned down by health and disability insurance companies because PICS is not widely viewed as a qualifying condition, and our team helps navigate this thorny issue.

We welcome people from all across the country whose lives have been affected by critical care. Some find their way to us after years struggling with symptoms they didn't realize were connected to an ICU stay, and some seek us out immediately after discharge, referred by critical care doctors who understand the need for follow-up. Given the evolution in critical care treatment over the years, we see varying degrees of PICS, often depending on how recently a patient was in the ICU—though that is not a hard-and-fast indicator. Our patients at the Recovery Center are all invited to attend our weekly ICU survivors' support group. We have now expanded its format to address the extensive needs of COVID long-haulers and their families. These survivors, numbering in the tens of millions around the world, experience the effects of COVID-19 weeks and months after the initial infection, referred to as Long COVID, or post-acute sequelae of SARS-CoV-2 infection (PASC), or post-acute COVID syndrome (PACS). The most common symptoms seem to be brain fog, exhaustion, shortness of breath, muscle weakness, diarrhea, and fluid retention (though there are many others), and these can impact people's ability to resume former activities and may prevent them from returning to work.

Long-hauler Heidi Ross spoke to our support group four months into her struggle with Long COVID and described her extreme fatigue, heavy legs, and difficulties with concentration. "On bad days, I will not only forget conversations or forget that I had conversations, but even as I'm having them, I will realize that I'm forgetting what we just said. I've come to really appreciate the days when that's not happening." While some long-haulers spent time in an ICU, others—such as Heidi—had a mild case of coronavirus and recuperated at home. The needs of long-haulers and ICU survivors clearly overlap: they both must have validation, support, and access to rehabilitation.

• • •

At a recent support group meeting, one of the newcomers, Rich, was quiet and sat with his head down, but when longtime attendee Tommy included him in the discussion, Rich lit up. He was still struggling with his memory after almost dying in an ICU far from his home. A computer programmer, he and his wife, Danielle, have three young kids. His family was struggling financially—Rich was laid off from his job when it became apparent that he just didn't understand the work anymore. Danielle commented that Rich seemed overwhelmed by anxiety and depression. But for two hours every week, he felt supported and understood. Joining the group, he said, was the best thing that had happened to him since his illness. "I feel like I belong here. You guys understand me."

Others nodded. It's something we hear frequently. Our survivors have often had their struggles dismissed by everyone from medical professionals to close friends and spouses. They feel misunderstood and isolated on top of everything else they are going through. For many, finally being heard, being seen and validated, is an enormous relief. Jean, who was using Zoom to connect from Virginia, described the frustration of people not taking her illness seriously. She started crying and apologized. "Go right ahead," said Sarah Beth. "That's what we're here for."

Audun Huslid found his way to our support group after reading about delirium in a magazine. Before that, he had spent four years looking for answers, trying to understand what had happened to him after his critical illness. He told me, "I wish my right hand were cut off so that people would know immediately that there's something wrong with me. Instead they look at me funny and wonder what my problem is." Audun was an investment banker on Wall Street but hasn't worked since his hospital discharge. He says he doesn't know who he is anymore. "The wheel I need to move forward is the wheel that's actually missing."

The types of disabilities that arise during critical care can disrupt the very core of a person's identity, their personhood. The acquired dementia we often see is perhaps the most obvious example of this as it can sever people's ability to interact and connect and may disrupt their sense of self. To support survivors of critical illness, we need to recognize that they carry their past stories and experiences into their present lives, and give them confidence that they are fully seen as a whole person.

Steve Edmonson and Lamar Hill, regulars at our support group meetings, are both former professional musicians who survived sepsis, only to find that they no longer even wanted to listen to music, much less play their instruments. Steve was a jazz and blues guitarist with the Dynatones in the nineties and then with the Jackie Payne Steve Edmonson Band from 2001 until his ICU admission in 2010. After his discharge, he told his wife, Judy, "I woke up a different person, one I don't particularly like." A key part of him had disappeared, but for years his doctors told him there was nothing wrong and nothing to be done. Music was Lamar's life, too. He played piano, drums, and guitar for legends such as Doc Watson, Ray Charles, and the Everly Brothers. Lamar had written to me, "The ICU took music completely out of me. It's gone. Vanished. The loss is a real mystery to me. It's part cognitive and part emotional and appears permanent." It was completely demoralizing for Lamar.

Both men came to our center desperate for help, and through many months of work with our team and encouragement from support group members, they are beginning to find their way forward. Steve and Lamar have become close, talking to each other at length, independent of the group sessions. Steve updated me: "I've been trying to get more comfortable just listening to music, and I find that I have been able to enjoy it!" We hope that in time he will be able to play his guitar again. For Lamar, music is not yet back in his life, and we continue to explore ways to help him with this. For sure, the support group—and his friendship with Steve—remains a positive for him.

Support groups create a safe space for shared experience, and more acute-care hospitals are beginning to focus on the aftercare of their critical illness survivors, providing them with such groups as a form of rehab and recovery, just as they do for patients surviving cancer and traumatic brain injury. The first historical record of such a group for intensive care patients was that run in 1992 by Christina Jones, of ICU diary fame, out of Whiston Hospital in the UK. Dr. Jones was hired early in her career by Dr. Richard Griffiths to study critical care patient outcomes and saw a real need for patients and families to understand that others were going through the same experiences. Originally, she set up a monthly meeting at the hospital, but no one showed up. She realized that many survivors were scared to return to the scene of their near-death experiences, so she arranged a meeting at a local pub. A crowd of people arrived, eager to talk over pints of ale. Dr. Jones laughingly explained, "As odd and British as it sounds, the first ICU survivors' support group was birthed over beer in a pub in Liverpool!"

Another pioneer at the grassroots level of ICU recovery groups was Eileen Rubin, who was just thirty-three and a newly minted lawyer in Chicago in 1994 when she got ARDS from a bacterial infection. She spent over sixty days in the hospital, had to wear diapers, lost 20 percent of her body weight, had five chest tubes inserted because of burst and collapsed lungs, and finally left the hospital in a wheelchair. Five years later, she founded the ARDS Foundation, the first survivor interest group in the United States for this common ICU illness that most people have never heard of. Her goal has been to educate the public about ARDS and to provide emotional support and practical resources for survivors, who often live with PICS, and their families. She told me, "There was nothing like it out there, and immediately people started contacting us from all over the world, hungry for information, hungry to share."

Whenever I attend a support group at our ICU Recovery Center, I notice the power of story both for our survivors, and their families, and for us, the medical professionals. This is a safe space where the survivors have the floor to say what they want about their illness and how it affects them, and in the telling to make sense of it. As a physician, I am there to listen and learn. I am reminded of narrative medicine, a relatively new field that integrates evidence-based medicine with story-based medicine to enhance patient-physician interactions. As Dr. Rita Charon, one of the field's pioneers, states, these connections are not "bureaucratic or technical encounters, but creative, singular, exposing human experiences." Narrative medicine strives to put the patient in charge of his own illness by recounting his story to a doctor instead of having to respond to a barrage of questions. In narrative medicine classes at medical schools, students are taught the benefits of bringing skills from reading literature to patient interactions as they look for patterns, themes, beginnings, middles, and ends. I was pleased to invite Dr. Hedy Wald from Brown University for a grand rounds talk on the possibilities for narrative and reflective writing to humanize our patient experiences, and our students now have multiple opportunities to explore narrative medicine in various areas of their curriculum. The practice has an intentionality that helps budding physicians as well as gray-haired ones such as myself process our patient experiences through reflection and writing.

• • •

The other day a new group attendee, Carol Billian, came from Baltimore and shared her story. Her life—like those of so many of the survivors present—had changed in hours. One moment she was discussing dinner plans, the next she was on the floor of her home with a ruptured colon and all her organs shutting down. Carol ended up in the ICU on life support, and when she was discharged to her mother's house four months later, she couldn't remember her own birthday. When she tried to resume her responsibilities of looking after the family real estate business, she didn't even know how to turn on her computer. She told the group, "I slid into depression, couldn't carry on my former life, and believe I am a textbook case of PICS."

Her fellow survivors listened and nodded as she described her terror at waking up in the ICU with no recollection of how she got there. They all knew that feeling, too. I looked at the faces of the people sitting around the conference table and on Zoom—Rich, Sarah Beth, Lovemore, Tommy, Steve, and many others. They had all gone through so much, yet here they were welcoming another survivor into their midst, ready to listen and share and help as much as they could. Carol was now one of them. The hell of critical illness had consumed her and she had survived and had a story to tell. There was room at their table for her. I could see the healing in that.

Something else struck me about Carol's story. It seemed that her recovery was much better than that of some of our longtime attendees. Less than two years after her ICU discharge, she was back in charge of the family business. She lived independently and was traveling by plane again. With her permission I tracked down her doctors at the community hospital near Baltimore where she received her treatment and, to my delight, learned that the standard care there was low sedation and early mobility and all the other elements of the bundle. Dr. Linda Barr, Carol's intensivist, told me, "Here at St. Joe's we are big on the A2F bundle!" So there was a reason that she was doing so well so soon after her ICU stay.

However, even with that treatment, Carol had suffered obvious cognitive impairment. I wondered how her brain had managed to regain some of this lost ground. When I asked Carol, she was thrilled and said, "Oh, so you want to hear about my brain games?" Frightened by her new deficiencies, she self-prescribed a daily program of ninety minutes of brain exercises. "I've done a mixture of word and number games, about forty-five minutes each, every day for the past twelve weeks." She was relentless and determined and, after diligently following this regimen, found that she was able to return to work. Just a week after her visit to our CIBS Center, she treated herself to a new laptop, backed up her old computer, transferred the files over, and was off and running on her new machine. She was elated and wrote to me, "I just danced a jig!" The brain training paid off.

• • •

A few years ago, I was in Tel Aviv, Israel, for their national critical care congress and, while traveling, immersed myself in *Thinking, Fast and Slow* by Israeli psychologist and economist Daniel Kahneman. In his fascinating book, he outlines two kinds of thinking: System 1 is quick, efficient, and concrete (and was a large part of Malcolm Gladwell's *Blink*), while System 2 is slower, led by deliberation and logic. The more I read, the more I became convinced that the predominant cognitive disabilities of so many of our ICU survivors fell into the System 2 category. As Kahneman explains, we use System 1 thinking when we are on autopilot, driving down the street, listening to our kids in the back seat, and changing the radio station. When it's time to turn left into traffic, we use System 2 thinking to override System 1 as we pause and map out a plan to navigate across lanes safely. It seemed to me that while survivors could still handle tasks that involved the instinctual and subconscious thoughts that dominate most people's thinking, the slower, deeper System 2 thinking was almost impossible for them. I was sure it wasn't a coincidence that many of our survivors had experienced multiple car accidents since their hospital discharges.

At around the same time, I started to read about neuroplasticity, the brain's capacity to reorganize itself by forming new neural connections. I found it especially interesting that the brain could adapt and compensate for injury and disease. In medical school at Tulane, I was taught that the brain could not regenerate and heal, that it was rigidly hardwired, and I'm sure that my cherished *Principles of Neural Science* from back then would have supported this thinking. If neurons died, they were gone. However, in the mid-1980s neuroscientists Dr. Jon Kaas at Vanderbilt University, Dr. Michael Merzenich at the University of California, San Francisco, and Dr. Edward Taub from the University of Alabama, among others, started to challenge this viewpoint through animal studies, and the field of neuroplasticity was born. In experiments in which strokes were induced to cause one-sided paralysis in rodents and primates, the animals learned not to use, for example, their left side. Their brain started to perform all tasks with the right side of the body, losing the left side forever. However, when Kaas, Merzenich, and Taub temporarily restricted the use of the animals' still-functioning limbs (on the right side) with various immobilization techniques, they didn't develop this "learned non-use." Once the inflammation had settled and the brain had started to repair, the animals were allowed to move freely, and the scientists discovered that the brain could rewire itself and make new connections to start using the left side of the body again. The brains of these animals exhibited unequivocal neuroplasticity.

After reading more about this work in Dr. Norman Doidge's book *The Brain That Changes Itself*, I started to see possibilities for our survivors. What if their brain could adapt and repair itself after the damage wrought during their ICU stay? I tracked down Dr. Doidge, and he invited me to the University of Alabama at Birmingham for the Neuroplasticity and Healing Summit with Dr. Merzenich, Dr. Taub, and the Dalai Lama, who is fascinated by the effects of meditation on the brain. I went to Alabama eager to listen to experts in neuroscience, an area of medicine so connected to my own work on delirium, and one in which I had much to learn. I had read the Dalai Lama's teaching on meditation several years earlier, and it intrigued me. He likened life to a river in which we are able to stop the flow and remain present in still water. I had taken to meditation at home and brought his teaching to my bedside practice to help my often anxious patients and their families stay in the moment and resist the temptation to live in either the past or the future.

Perhaps the most instructive portion of the program for me was the conversation about constraint-induced therapy (CIT), an approach to brain rehabilitation pioneered by our host, Dr. Taub. The human application of the early animal work, CIT has been developed by Taub to help rewire the brains of humans to optimize recovery from traumatic brain injury, strokes, brain tumors, and even multiple sclerosis. Through his work, thousands of people have improved their brain functioning after injuries. As I listened, I wondered if these cognitive rehabilitation concepts might be useful to improve recovery from the post-ICU dementia suffered by millions of people around the world.

Since then we have been working on a multifold approach at the CIBS Center to help our patients with PICS regain their brain function. We have used exercises to rehabilitate the brain's ability to perform executive tasks, which are so often impaired after the ICU. Initially we used a program called Goal Management Training (GMT), developed by Dr. Brian Levine from the University of Toronto, the purpose of which is to improve a person's executive function by helping them learn to be reflective—to "stop and think" about consequences of decisions before making them. The patient divides tasks into manageable units, which I like to call bite-size morsels, to increase the likelihood of completion. We have also worked with a computerized version of GMT, enabling many people to work on the program more repetitively and allowing us to track their compliance.

Currently, we are taking advantage of recent developments in neuroscience and technology to bring cognitive rehabilitation to more of our survivors. We are undertaking research in this area funded by the Department of Veterans Affairs, and Dr. Michael Merzenich's BrainHQ cognitive exercises will be used in an upcoming clinical trial for ICU survivors. We are also leveraging advances by neuroscientist Dr. Adam Gazzaley, from the University of California, San Francisco, and the company Akili, who together developed the first-ever FDA-approved video game that can be prescribed for cognitive rehabilitation. We are employing their exciting and highly adaptive computerized games in some of our cognitive rebuilding studies, too. Our hope is that these investigations will show that brain-training exercises can translate into real gains in the daily lives of our ICU survivors. If we can teach their System 2 thinking to recognize situations where it should take over from System 1 thinking, we can facilitate such things as reading, operating a spreadsheet of real estate deals, and writing and playing music.

To shape our treatment and rehabilitation approaches in the future, we are determining the exact nature of acquired dementia after critical illness. Now included in the family of Alzheimer's Disease and Related Dementias (ADRDs), we know it can intrude into people's lives within a single ICU stay. Unlike a stroke or TBI, it is not immediately visible as a "macro" injury on a brain CT or MRI. Instead, patients develop a diffuse sort of "micro" injury arising from millions and millions of lost and damaged neurons, the cells that transmit nerve impulses in the brain, and glial cells, the cells that create a latticework of support for neurons. As we saw in our VISIONS study, these changes to the brain show up months later, as a loss of brain tissue.

We are now funded by the NIH's Aging Institute to establish a brain repository. Dr. Mayur Patel, a trauma surgeon, and Dr. Angela Jefferson, a clinical neuropsychologist, both in the CIBS Center, and I partnered with a Rush University team of neuroscientists to carry out our BRAIN-2 study. In this investigation, we will examine brains at a cellular level for many of the different conditions that can result in the dementia that ICU survivors struggle with: we will look for Alzheimer's, different types of strokes, Lewy bodies, and CTE, as well as evidence of dying and dead brain cells and disruption of their means of communication. We hope our discoveries will shape prevention programs and cognitive rehabilitation going forward.

• • •

The three-pound human brain is extraordinary. It has 80 billion to 1 quadrillion neurons, each with ten to fifteen thousand connections to other brain cells. That is up to between 100 trillion and 1,000 trillion synapses that are constantly being modified every second of every day.

Glial cells, namely microglia and astrocytes, are looking more and more like central figures in the story of our brain's well-being. Microglia, in particular, are recognized as regulating inflammation in the brain. Astrocytes, long thought of as the glue that holds the brain together, are known to be critical to maintain the blood-brain barrier, regulate immune responses, and contribute to the health and growth of neurons. The complex interplay between all of these cell types will be the key to unlocking patients' brain recovery after injury. This potential for rebuilding gives me great hope.

I was especially interested in survivor Carol Billian's experience with her self-imposed brain training, as it seemed to be an example of neuroplasticity in action. For three months she pushed herself to work through the exercises. She told me it felt like crawling out of a deep trench that had prevented her from seeing and understanding things around her. Was it possible that Carol's exercises had grown new brain tissue?

In 2006, Dr. Eleanor Maguire and her colleagues, neuroscientists at University College London, did a thought-provoking experiment in which they studied the gray matter volume in the hippocampus of licensed taxi drivers and compared it to that of a control group of bus drivers in London. To obtain their full "green badge" license, the taxi drivers must memorize a dizzyingly complex map of more than 25,000 streets (many of which are one-way), along with the locations of thousands of places of interest within a six-mile radius of Charing Cross railway station. This training, known as acquiring the Knowledge, typically takes between three and four years. Taxi drivers navigate the city's thousands of streets in many and diverse ways. In contrast, London bus drivers are fully approved after just six weeks of training and adhere to the strict routes assigned to them, over and over without deviation. While there are some fine details to this study, the authors found through MRI imaging that compared to the bus drivers, the taxi drivers had significantly increased gray matter in the posterior hippocampus, a structure critical to the formation of new memories. Dr. Maguire showed clearly how the day-to-day activity of our minds can lead to new connections and increased structural volume in the brain. To use the analogy of London's city map, the brain could be building more streets (neurogenesis), connecting existing ones (synaptogenesis), or building infrastructure (proliferation of glial cells). To some extent, much of this neuroplasticity must have occurred inside Carol's brain.

The question now is how we best apply this knowledge on a large scale through cognitive rehabilitation to millions of suffering ICU survivors, such as Carol, who want their brains back.

• • •

Just like the Lansing family, many of our critical care survivors are in need of mental health counseling to help with anxiety, depression, and PTSD.

Kyle Mullicane, my patient with pancreatitis and catatonia, whose delirium brought him face-to-face with a black jaguar, is still learning to cope. He believes that therapy is enabling him to understand that when the wild cat does show up, it isn't real. Mental health counseling is guiding him through his vulnerability, helping him figure out a way forward. He and his wife, Katie, believe that his ICU diary with videos and notes from his stay has helped him to process and understand a lot of what happened to him while he was sedated. He has watched videos of himself in his ICU bed talking with family members and friends, and learned that nothing strange or nefarious was going on. The world of distorted visions he lived in throughout his stay was just that: a twisted reality in his brain.

I reconnected with Dr. Christina Jones, pioneer of ICU diaries, during the height of the COVID-19 pandemic, where she spoke to me from retirement at her home on the coast of Wales. I could hear the seagulls in the background. She explained that she conceived of the diary as a way to help fill in the blanks for those who struggle to remember their ICU stay or for those with false memories, often caused by delirium.

As we were talking, she paused, then said, "I'd like to tell you about one particular lad. He was eighteen and had survived a traumatic spinal cord injury. As part of his therapy, he transitioned from a regular bed into a spinal bed that holds the body in an oddly stiff position. When I showed him his diary with pictures that I'd taken of the bed, he exclaimed, 'Ahh, that explains everything.' It turned out he had suffered horrible nightmares about being trapped in the film *The Matrix*. Now he knew exactly where that nightmare had come from. For some people, a single photograph can unlock everything."

As our patients reenter their lives, our aim is to support them every step of the way. My patient Todd Bowlin almost died from sepsis stemming from sinusitis. He needed help to return to his job on a farm, as a jack-of-all-trades as Lydia, his wife, puts it. Even though he received early exercise and mobility interventions, walking the length of the ICU hall with his young sons skipping at his side, he still experienced muscle loss during his stay. Minutes of activity now left him completely winded. Studies show that mechanically ventilated patients lose nearly 20 percent of their muscle mass during the first ICU week, and they can rapidly age into frailty, as assessed by the Clinical Frailty Scale, based on factors including physical activity, cognition, and dependence on others for day-to-day living. Physical impairments that usually take years to develop may come on within days during an ICU stay, even for younger patients such as Todd.

Post-ICU care is crucial if recovery is to be possible. Soon after discharge, we arranged for physical therapy sessions for Todd in his home so that he could strengthen and condition his weakened muscles. Next, the therapist went to the farm with him to assess the requirements of his job and had him work on exercises with practical applications, such as climbing in and out of his tractor over and over, or carrying heavy bundles of rope. When it became clear that Todd needed cognitive rehab, too, an occupational therapist worked with him. His memory wasn't what it used to be, and he had trouble grasping the correct sequencing to get tasks done. Again, the therapist came to his home and to the farm to understand what would be most helpful for Todd. She assisted him with learning to clock in at work, how to use the computer, and to develop systems that could jog his memory. When I checked in with him recently, just over a year after his discharge, he had returned to work full-time and felt that he was well on his way to being back to where he was before.

It's a relief to see that this kind of personalized care after critical illness makes a huge difference in our patients' recovery and enables them to transition back to their former lives. Todd is one of the fortunate ones. In an analysis of fifty-two studies of over ten thousand previously employed ICU survivors, 40 percent were unemployed one year after their hospital discharge, while 33 percent were jobless five years after discharge. In addition, after initially returning to work, up to 36 percent experienced subsequent job loss, 66 percent had an occupation change, and as many as 84 percent experienced a worsening employment status such as fewer work hours. These figures and those from other studies highlight both the devastating consequences of critical care that survivors must grapple with, and the need for supportive aftercare to help them get back on their feet. The benefits of regaining mastery of a former job are not only financial, though that is obviously important. When our survivors can return to activities they once enjoyed, they reclaim a sense of self-worth, dignity, independence, identity, and structure, and this promotes their emotional and psychological well-being. Everyone benefits.

• • •

The new patient in Bed 6 in the Veterans Affairs ICU looked as if he were dozing, an extra blanket wrapped around his shoulders. No one seemed to be with him, no family photos were on the bedside table, but maybe someone would come in to see him later in the day. I made a note in his chart to find out about family and to read through the record. I saw that he was in prison a year earlier, that his blood sugar and cholesterol were both too high, and his sodium was too low. As I approached the bed, he opened his eyes and blinked up at me.

"Good morning, Mr. Lewis! I'm Dr. Ely, and I'm here to care for you today."

His glance slid sideways. I started right in to test him for delirium, explaining what I was doing. "Squeeze my hand every time you hear me say the letter *A*, and if you hear me say a different letter, don't squeeze. Ready?"

He nodded, his breathing tube moving up and down.

"I'm sorry. We'll make this easy on you."

He shrugged.

"A." Firm squeeze. *"B."* Nothing. *"R."* Nothing. *"A."* Nothing. I continued saying the letters in *ABRACADABRA*, and Mr. Lewis squirmed a little, looking straight at me, but did not respond. He was awake and conscious, but completely unable to remain attentive.

After finishing my exam, I told the team that he had hypoactive delirium, the quiet kind that can manifest as sluggishness and apathy and is missed 75 percent of the time when not objectively monitored with a delirium tool. I thought how easy it would be to dismiss him as an uncooperative patient. He had missed two dialysis sessions and was fluid overloaded—no wonder his sodium levels were dangerously low, which could help to explain his delirium. Now he was irritated to find himself back in the ICU. I wondered if, when I was younger, I might have just assumed he was being belligerent.

"What do we know about his missed sessions?" I asked. "Could he not get here? Can we consult our team's social worker?"

"We already did," said a young doctor. "Something to do with the police. They came to look for him at the hospital the last time he was here."

That might explain things. I could imagine that a person would be reluctant to go to a dialysis appointment if he was concerned about running into law enforcement there. And now Mr. Lewis was critically ill.

"Let me know when the social worker is here, okay?" I asked. "I'd like to be a part of that conversation."

I was pleased that the residents had already thought to involve a social worker and were aware that when we treat a patient, we must also address the outside factors that lead to illness and injury. Patients' circumstances affect their health, and their ability to access care. We think of these as upstream factors.

Social determinants of health are the conditions in places where people live, work, go to school, and play that affect a vast range of risks and outcomes. Especially important factors are the standard of housing, education levels, community support, access to health insurance and medical care, availability of public transportation, levels of poverty, employment, and violence.

As a teenager I had noticed that the farm pickers I worked with did not go to see doctors regularly, though I could not have listed the reasons why. Now I understand that they did not have health insurance. They were paid daily and could not afford to take time off to see a doctor, or to stay home and be sick.

The pickers' circumstances are reflected in varying ways across our country, where people live in poverty without access to basic health care, with more fast-food than grocery stores in their neighborhoods, and without parks or green spaces for exercise. Reading my Vanderbilt colleague Dr. Jonathan Metzl's work on ways we, as a medical community, must become better engaged with the prevalence of social injustice and racism, I found the science illuminating. Epigenetics research—the study of how our behavior and environment change the way our genes work—demonstrates that high-stress, resource-poor conditions can create risk factors for diseases including cancer, heart disease, and diabetes. Neuroscientists have found that social exclusion, poverty, and chronic stress can negatively impact brain development and can lead to mental health disorders, and economists have shown that when people with low income move into safer, wealthier areas they have lower rates of diabetes, obesity, and depression.

While I have grown better at following my patients into their lives after discharge, their downstream recovery, I know I still need to look upstream more. Only then will I see the whole picture, the whole human. What if we in the ICU infused our clinical practice (and medical education) with awareness of the myriad life realities affecting patient compliance, acquisition of disease, and access to affordable health care? During COVID, I—and so many others in health care—were struck by the disproportionate number of Black and Hispanic Americans who both caught coronavirus and who died from it compared with white Americans. The pandemic held up a magnifying glass and highlighted disparities both within society and the health-care system. It is not random that many Hispanic workers, dependent on each day's wages and thus unable to take time off work if ill, and sometimes living in tight quarters, acquired high rates of COVID-19 infection and filled our ICUs. Many have devoted families at home, yet when we opened our hospital to visitation, their loved ones were often not able to be at the bedside. Their upstream circumstances dictated that they did not have childcare or could not skip work for fear of missing a paycheck, losing a job, and then, potentially, their home.

Fred Reyes was admitted to our COVID-ICU when he went down with ARDS from coronavirus. Due to the hospital's visitation policy, his wife, Sharon, was unable to visit, and Fred felt profoundly alone. Intubated and sedated on the ventilator, he asked for her every day, writing her name on a whiteboard. Sharon was first in line when visitation opened again. "I just wanted to be with him, cheering him on, encouraging him, touching him. Being helpless and dependent is the opposite of his personality, and us being separated is the opposite of our relationship."

After weeks of a profoundly complicated stay, Fred survived. He has ongoing PICS-related muscle and nerve problems in his legs and can't think the way he used to. The loss of his job as a camp director has contributed to depression. But when I visited him in the rehabilitation hospital, it seemed that what had frightened and upset him the most during his stay was his loss of agency. He told me about growing up in the Southwest and how his family experienced prejudice at every turn. "We had no voice and learned to fight for our freedom and dignity. That's where I come from." And his ICU experience had brought all this back to him, magnifying his fear and loneliness. Even with compassionate nurses, he had felt silenced by his illness, and afraid. As I looked him in the eyes, I knew I had to face some important truths about humanness, disparity, and our society. Everyone's experience of critical illness was unique, made up of who each person is. And caregivers had to be attentive to each story. We had to lift our gaze to see all our patients.

• • •

Recently, I was fortunate enough to connect with author and poet Guy Johnson, son of Dr. Maya Angelou. Her voice had echoed in my mind over the decades since I cared for her at Wake Forest Medical Center, when she was preparing her poem "On the Pulse of Morning." I was excited to speak with Mr. Johnson. When asked what it was like to grow up in the shadow of his mother, he responded, "I grew up in her light. Sometimes I wasn't worthy of it, but it has always been an experience that expanded me." I sensed this graciousness, this wise humility, when we spoke. I told him, with a schoolboy's enthusiasm, about the way his mother's words had reached me and struck a chord. He told me, "My mother always said she wrote from the Black perspective, but she aimed for the human heart."

We talked about the challenges that racial tensions bring up for society and individuals, and the way the pandemic had shown that some communities are more vulnerable than others. It made me stop and think about how I could change my work as a doctor for the better, and I shared this with him. Mr. Johnson seemed to understand and told me of the need for society to embrace a spirit of "cultural empathy."

As Mr. Johnson spoke, I was intrigued by his words. I could see how it would be better for my patients if I developed a heightened awareness of their cultures, in addition to getting to know them as individuals. There was so much I wanted to know about him, his life. It made me think, "What if I were meeting him as a patient in my ICU? Would I have so many questions?" The depersonalization chamber sprang to mind.

A person's cultural background is one of the many things that gets stripped away in the stressful setting of the ICU. But it shouldn't. It mustn't. So much makes up each complicated, wonderful human being looking for healing. Cultural empathy embraces a sense of equity, equality, respect, and love. The more I understand and incorporate cultural empathy into my bedside practice as a physician, the better I can care for my patients both in and beyond the ICU. The more I will be able to say, "I see you."

Chapter 12

End-of-Life Care in the ICU—Patient and Family Wishes Can Come True

So few grains of happiness
measured against all the dark
and still the scales balance.

—Jane Hirshfield, "The Weighing"

WHILE MAKING ROUNDS IN our Veterans Affairs ICU in the spring of 2020, I had the honor of meeting retired US army colonel Victor Correa, a recipient of the Soldier's Medal and the Purple Heart, awarded for risking his life for others by crawling through fire, smoke, and the debris of an exploded plane at the Pentagon on 9/11. On that day, he was so bewildered by all the death and destruction that, after carrying many others to safety, he trudged the long miles home to his house in Arlington, covered in blood. Only when he stopped moving did he discover he had a dislocated hip. As I stood at his bedside, he was on a ventilator. Lymphoma had riddled his body, and pneumonia filled his lungs. This American hero knew he didn't have long to live. He was not hoping for a miracle cure, just to be taken off the ventilator so he could speak with his wife, Sergeant First Class Oretta Correa, and their five children. He needed to say his goodbyes, and he had written instructions for me on his whiteboard: "Pain 4 or 5 but must stay clear for family."

Despite our best efforts, depending on the patient, the severity of illness, and admission diagnosis, between 10 percent and 30 percent of people who come into our ICU with critical illness will die there. One in five deaths in the United States occurs in a critical care bed— and when it becomes clear to the medical team that we cannot save a patient's life, our thoughts and actions must turn from cure to comfort. It becomes time to focus not on what's the matter *with* the patient, but what matters *to* the patient. I have found that this switch of the preposition serves extremely well for patients and families to open a gateway of communication and sharing. Things get personal immediately. We can't address patients' wishes about dying unless we first ask what those wishes are. What's more, we can't ask them their preferences if they are heavily sedated or profoundly delirious.

In the documentary *Oliver Sacks: His Own Life*, physician and author Dr. Danielle Ofri asks the great neurologist how his experiences of being a patient changed him as a person and a doctor.

Sacks recalls undergoing orthopedic surgery. "I found the inability to communicate my feelings to the surgeon almost worse than what was happening with the leg. . . . [I] needed someone to listen and someone to be empathic." Giving patients the opportunity to express their needs is key, especially at the end of life.

Colonel Correa continued to let me know his wishes, writing, "Get out of bed. Think better. Talk to family." As his physician, it was vital that I do everything I could to honor this, so I needed to focus on managing his pain, dyspnea (shortness of breath), anxiety, and delirium. Over the next twenty-four hours, we worked hard to lessen the fluid in his lungs to take him safely off the ventilator. We removed him completely from sedation, and to help with his pain and anxiety, I increased his morphine doses just enough to keep him comfortable. He had made it clear that he wanted his mind to be unclouded so he could speak with his wife and children. To reduce the likelihood of delirium further, his nurses and I heaved him out of bed and into a chair. Then we groomed his beard and got him ready to see his family.

We were under strict COVID-19 isolation, but he was negative for the virus. Through close communication with our hospital leadership, we received permission to have his loved ones at his bedside. First Oretta made her way to him, and a smile spread across his face. Next, their eldest daughter, Lydia, surprised him, standing in the doorway to his room. He looked as if he might try to scramble out of his chair to hug her. "Daddy, you look so handsome." He beamed and slowly said, "I know I do." He had a mischievous air.

Lydia hurried over to me, outside his room, and said, "Did you see? When I walked in, he wriggled up in the chair." She hadn't expected her father to be conscious for his goodbyes, and I saw how much it meant to her that he was. She turned and headed back into his room. I popped my head around the door a little later; all his children were sitting together, talking.

Over the next week, his family sat with him, chatting, telling him whatever was in their hearts and reminiscing about his life—the big 9/11 events, of course, yet with his favorite 1980s music playing in the background, I heard stories about the small things, too, his everyday kindnesses that had woven a thread through their lives. When he could no longer speak, he scribbled, "Peace, love u, read to me," to Oretta. The palliative care team and the chaplain worked together to address his suffering, including his spiritual needs through praying Psalm 91 and Isaiah 12 with him and Oretta as they requested.

In his final days, Colonel Correa's pain and discomfort increased and we turned up his morphine. With all their words for him expressed, Oretta and the children—Lydia, Victor, Andrea, Victoria, and Jose—held his hands as he took his last breath. At just that moment, Oretta lifted her head to look at the clock and exclaimed, "Oh, it's 9:11." And so it was. On the dot.

• • •

As a young doctor, I thought of death in the ICU as a form of failure. I didn't like to think too much about that stack of index cards of patients who didn't make it. Whenever death occurred, I felt a sense of nihilism. It festered deep inside, revealing itself when things seemed futile. I knew that each person came to my ICU with the hope of more life; no one arrived there planning to die, yet frequently the scales tilted irrevocably toward death. And when we couldn't save the person, I had seen death as defeat. On occasion, dying patients were sent to us by physicians in other parts of the hospital, as if we could work a special kind of magic that would defy the evidence in their medical charts. This always saddened me, and the nihilism would simmer to the surface again. I no longer feel this way. Now I realize that often my referring colleagues are hoping their patient might have a little more time with a loved one. I have learned that my energy is best spent helping a patient and his family navigate the end-of-life stages. Often that means talking through the decision to withhold or withdraw life-sustaining therapies that are no longer indicated when taking an honest look at the particulars of a patient's medical condition.

When it becomes evident that a patient in my care will die, I no longer think, "There's nothing more I can do." While that may technically be true with regard to sustaining life, I can still tend to my patients in many ways while they are dying. With Colonel Correa, we worked on his medical needs in a way that met his emotional wishes; calibrating his pain medication to keep his mind sharp; watching and counting his breaths to ensure he wasn't feeling a drowning sensation after extubation; monitoring him for delirium; and working with the palliative care team. Much of this happened in the background so he and his family could enjoy their final days together. I have come to see this as the opposite of failure.

• • •

Mrs. Barberousse was in the hospital receiving antibiotics for pneumonia when she suddenly flipped into an irregular heart rhythm called atrial fibrillation. Her heart raced so fast that fluid surged into her lungs like a flash flood, and she started to struggle to breathe. With widely metastatic breast cancer that had spread to her lungs, bones, and brain, she had a Do Not Resuscitate order in her chart, and up in the ICU we questioned whether we should receive her as a transfer.

"There is nothing we can do for her," said another doctor, an echo of my own attitude from some years earlier. "She would just be coming here to die."

But the critical care fellow argued to admit her. I immediately backed his decision, and Mrs. Barberousse was transferred to our ICU service. We fitted her with a noninvasive breathing mask called BiPAP. This soon relieved her breathing and allowed time for heart rate medications and fluid pills to work. It became obvious that our patient would not be dying that very night, but we also knew she did not have much time left. This was the moment to focus on comfort. On what mattered to her. Our ICU team worked with Mrs. Barberousse and palliative care physicians to plan a comfortable dying process, and to ensure that she would receive helpful social services, including home hospice. As we talked, her eyes sparkled as she told us about her grandson's upcoming wedding. Being able to attend would clearly mean everything to her. We made sure to include this in our planning as Mrs. Barberousse left the ICU.

A couple of months later, I was in my office when I received a hand-addressed envelope in the mail. When I opened it, some photographs tumbled onto my desk. Wedding pictures. As I looked closely, there was Mrs. Barberousse, portable oxygen at her side, proudly standing next to her grinning grandson and his new bride. Her final wish. She had made it.

• • •

For the past ten years, I have spent time working in different regions of Haiti as part of global health initiatives. One of my most memorable opportunities was to participate in a project with Dr. Paul Farmer through Partners In Health (PIH) and their sister organization, Zanmi Lasante (ZL). Founded in 1987, PIH, a social justice nonprofit, brings high-quality health care to impoverished communities around the world and, in 2013, opened University Hospital of Mirebalais, a three-hundred-bed teaching facility, to provide care to the local area in central Haiti. Usually I work alongside the Haitian health teams in whatever capacity they feel I can be most helpful, but for this project, I was collaborating with them to establish state-of-the-art critical care in the world's first Black republic. I was part of a group of ICU doctors from various US-based hospitals spending monthlong shifts there to partner in building the program. Eventually it would be sustained by the Haitian nurses and physicians, many of whom had trained at the hospital, under the leadership of Dr. Carlos St. Cyr, the director of the ICU at Mirebalais.

On my first day, while rounding in the sizzling heat in the ICU, I stood with Dr. St. Cyr at the bedside of Mr. Tuff Domond, an emaciated man on a mechanical ventilator. Weeks earlier, while plowing a near-vertical hillside to plant corn for the coming year, somehow he had fallen, rolled, and smashed into a tree. Several farmers lifted his injured body into the back of a weathered wooden cart pulled by a donkey and brought him twelve miles along rocky dirt roads to the modern large hospital. To them it must have looked like a vision of hope.

I examined Mr. Domond carefully from head to toe and reviewed his records. He had suffered a displaced femur fracture during his fall and had quickly developed pneumonia. I thought this might have been initiated by the spread of a fat embolism—fat seeping from the marrow of his cracked thighbone into his blood vessels and then wreaking havoc in his lungs. Operating was judged too risky by the surgeons.

As I listened to the ventilator pushing air into his stiff chest, I was dismayed to see how thin he was. He was suffering the same muscle wasting that Richard Griffiths had described decades earlier in the UK, that Polly Bailey had seen in Joy Sundloff's body in Utah all those years before, and on down the line. I lifted his good leg and saw the outline of his femur. Gone were the lean muscles that had pushed him up the mountains at harvesttime. I wasn't sure he would ever walk— or work—again. How would Mr. Domond fare beyond the hospital, supposing the bone eventually mended, if he was too weak to get around or earn money?

The feelings of nihilism seethed again. What had at first seemed so exciting—expanding critical care and the A2F bundle into a country only nominally exposed to life-support technology—now seemed as if it might generate new problems for people who were already suffering. Dr. St. Cyr told me that Mr. Domond was surely one of the first patients in Haiti, if not the index patient, to develop PICS. Their country was still grappling with the ravages of a cholera outbreak, reintroduced a few years earlier, likely by a United Nations peacekeeping mission. I wondered if I would be complicit in another man-made problem here if the technology was introduced without the preparation to handle ICU survivors.

Later that morning we admitted a pregnant woman, Asmith Charles, from a nearby village. She was seizing due to advanced eclampsia, and we swiftly intubated her and placed her on one of our two remaining ventilators. I was starting to feel rattled, concerned about our capacity to handle these complicated patients and about what would happen if another showed up. It felt as if we were unleashing something that would be difficult to rein in, a Pandora's box of sorts.

"You know, for Mr. Domond," said Dr. St. Cyr, "it's not enough to simply give him the ventilator. We must figure out how to get him back home safely. Is that doable? And for Mrs. Charles, now that we have her stabilized, we must get that baby delivered today, or she's going to die."

He was right. We had to focus on the task at hand. Just as Paul Farmer and cofounder of PIH Ophelia Dahl had vowed, looking out across the countryside under the Haitian night skies wondering how they would move forward with such a Herculean task. As they gazed into the dark, they saw pockets of illumination from stoked fires—affirming the creole mantra *Kenbe fem*, "stand firm." The fires gave them strength. They assured each other their work would take shape one person at a time.

Mr. Domond did not survive, dying of sepsis-related complications in the hospital. To my surprise, his family brought the ICU team a bounteous feast of crispy grilled goat, fried plantains, and juicy mangoes to thank us for the days they had spent with him as he was dying, time they would never have had if not for the new critical care unit. Their radiant smiles reminded me again of the power of modern medical technology even when an ICU stay ended in death.

The sight of Mrs. Charles, alive and getting better with newborn Novindi nestled by her side, reaffirmed for me the value of working alongside my Haitian colleagues as a small cog in building sustainable critical care for the country. My role was to follow Dr. St. Cyr and his team's lead so they could implement the bundle, save lives, and get people back to working, raising families, and finding meaning. And, when death was imminent, to make sure that patients were supported and loved ones were near. I remembered that when Pandora opened the box, hope remained.

• • •

Not so many years ago, palliative care and critical care were often viewed as mutually exclusive: one aimed at helping people with dying while the other focused on extending life. Now, however, more and more ICU teams have come to value the role that palliative care can play in the critical care setting, and to understand that it is not only for when a patient is dying. We know now that palliative care should be considered based not on a patient's prognosis but on their needs. There are dying cancer patients whose suffering is well controlled while there are cured surgical ICU patients whose clinical needs are so complex that they need nuanced palliative care. The aim is to enhance the quality of life for people with serious illness, make their suffering more bearable, and improve their overall wellness—physical, emotional, spiritual, and social.

Our patient-centered and family-centered care helps provide this level of support and facilitates the integration of a patient's personal goals into medical treatment. When I combine intensive care with palliative care, I am giving my patients primary palliative care. In some cases, I consult with a board-certified palliative care team for additional help, and this is specialty palliative care. The two go hand in hand. It is important, though, for all ICU teams to embrace their key role in providing primary palliative care, as there are not enough specialists to tend to all the suffering we see. In some hospitals and in some regions of the world, there are none.

Over the years, I have evolved into a primary palliative care physician and have witnessed the serenity it brings to my patients and their families. Others within the critical care field have noticed this, too, and have generated a body of studies and scientific literature about letting people go and advancing our knowledge of the best practices of caring for dying people in the ICU. For example, in 2015, Dr. Charlie Sprung from Jerusalem and Dr. Christiane Hartog of Berlin led a large study of end-of-life practices around the world and, compared to fifteen years earlier, found marked increases in legislation, policies, bioethics courses, palliative care, and ethics consultations. Dr. Élie Azoulay from Paris proved the benefits of allowing family to be present during CPR, and Dr. Randy Curtis from Seattle developed metrics of the quality of dying and death. Drs. Jessica Zitter and Ira Byock focused beautifully on the existential needs of patients during palliative care, and Dr. Doug White from Pittsburgh developed family support interventions for the ICU.

One of the most influential experts in the critical care field is Canadian icon Dr. Deborah Cook. A professor in the Department of Medicine at McMaster University, she seeks through her research to improve clinical treatments for critically ill patients who are either fighting life-threatening illnesses or facing end-of-life situations. Early on in Deborah's career, senior physician leaders and department chairpersons told her that focusing on end of life was beneath her, was "soft science, unsuitable for a serious investigator, a dead end, and even unethical to study." This horrified and humiliated her, but she pressed forward anyway. Now Deborah's 3 Wishes Project helps physicians and family members carry out the personal wishes of dying patients. I have known Deborah for a long time and consider her a wise friend, generous with her knowledge. We caught up with each other as the pandemic increased its deadly grip. As with so many other physicians in end-of-life care, the year had been both exhausting and deeply meaningful for her.

Deborah grew up near Lake Ontario, enjoying a happy childhood, one filled with sports and good schooling. She continued her passion for sports at McMaster, studying physical education, but her job in the health sciences library led her to meet medical students, read medical textbooks, and discover her hidden vocation. Other than for two years of critical care training at Stanford, she has been at McMaster University ever since. At Stanford, she studied under the legendary bioethicist Dr. Ernlé Young, who underscored for her that "it's possible to marry physiology, great clinical care, and the scholarly science and ethics of end-of-life care."

In 2012, she organized a forum on the last hundred days of life at which Dr. Peter Singer, a professor of bioethics with a background in philosophy, gave the closing remarks. Known for his work on effective altruism, he called on the audience to stop talking and start doing. He asked all the attendees to come up with a practical application in their own work for bettering end-of-life care. And to stand up and tell everyone at the forum about it. Deborah was a little panicked by this, but from her words that day she created the 3 Wishes Project, a way to personalize death in the ICU, bring serenity to the final days of a patient's life, ease grieving for family members, and enable clinicians to develop a deeper sense of vocation.

During the first demonstration project in a twenty-one-bed ICU in Ontario, each family-patient-physician unit came up with at least three wishes honoring the patient, to be carried out before or after his death. Deborah told me of personalized word clouds printed to celebrate a patient's values. Sunflowers placed in tall vases at bedsides. Live music played. Pets brought in, dogs and rabbits and even a skunk. Pizza delivered. Tea parties. Video-call reunions. "These are acts of compassion from the clinician," Deborah said. "I teach the junior nurses or docs to go in there and have a conversation, ask the family open-ended questions. 'Can you tell me more about your mom?' 'Where did your uncle meet his partner?' You just start a conversation." From there, the wishes arise organically, and their fulfillment is set in motion.

The results were overwhelmingly favorable and inexpensive. Eliciting and granting wishes encouraged individualized end-of-life care and helped family members to create memories and closure in anticipation of death. For the ICU team, implementing the three wishes exemplified humanism in practice and reduced feelings of distress.

I've used a version of 3 Wishes many times at my own patients' bedsides. For the most part their last requests have been relatively easy to meet: a bite of vegetable samosa, a cold beer, reconnecting with an old friend, watching a beloved movie with a spouse. Once, we looked after a mailman whose family told us one of his biggest life accomplishments was overcoming his fear of dogs. His nurse suggested we put Bacchus, a pet-therapy yellow Lab, on his legs in his ICU bed. For days, despite our efforts, his heart had raced at 140 beats per minute, but soon after Bacchus's arrival, it lowered to the seventies with no other changes in his medical care. Bacchus, sensing his purpose, refused to leave the bed until the patient sauntered out of life later that night.

I have always been struck by how small most people's last requests are, yet how large in meaning. A hand tenderly grasped. Caring words exchanged. A cherished memory shared. The things that buoy our lives bring solace, too, in death and beyond.

• • •

Recently, I sat at the bedside of sixty-three-year-old Mr. Jimmie Johnson. It appeared to us he was dying, and in accordance with his wishes, we had just taken him off the ventilator as part of his palliative care plan. A few days earlier, we had admitted him to our ICU from a local prison, and the team's emphasis was on antibiotic choices, fluid management, and ventilator settings. But in the midst of the rush of trying to save his life, my gaze kept returning to the bright red, heavy metal cuffs shackling his left leg. I had seen this before with other patients from the prison, but this time it continued to bother me. I asked our team, "Why does a man this gravely ill, on a ventilator, clearly unable to do anyone harm, require shackles? Can't we take them off?" Through the residents' fatigued glares and foot tapping, I heard them mentally grumbling, "Dr. Ely is so easily distracted. Can't he stay focused?"

I asked the guard to unlock him. He refused. He had instructions to leave #358041 in chains. I faxed a medical order to the prison physician and warden instructing that the tonic I was prescribing for my patient was to have his cuffs removed. Within an hour, the red cuffs hung loosely from his bedpost, and his body was free. I won't ever forget the nod Mr. Johnson gave me as he gazed down and pulled his knees up toward his chest. It will compel me to act quicker next time I have an opportunity to help restore a patient's dignity.

Later, as I sat with Mr. Johnson, he talked and talked, his voice slow and soft. I wasn't sure how long he might live, but he was clear that he didn't want further interventions. He seemed content to share with me stories from his childhood, the big farm where he had grown up in rural Tennessee, its wraparound porch with rocking chairs. I watched his oxygen saturations and made him slow down when they dipped too low. "There was a swimming hole, fishing hole, whatever you want to call it, but most of all, it had horses." He smiled. "I loved to ride horses. I'd sneak off and go ride after school and get in trouble mostly every day because I was late for dinner." His gaze was distant as he remembered, and I could see that farm, the horses, too. I wondered about his family now.

For several days, Philip Wilson, one of our medical students, worked to restore visitation rights for Jimmie's sister, Johnnie Blackwell, so that she could come see him. For the first time in years, they were able to hug, and they sat in his room together on her birthday, holding hands. It was Halloween. Johnnie giggled as stories spilled out of her. "When Jimmie was sixteen, he got a car from our grandfather, and from then on he was gone. He found a girl to marry, and by seventeen, he had his first daughter, Shatika. She was born on April Fools' Day!" They grinned at each other, with many more tales to recount. I am certain that nothing did more to mitigate the dying Jimmie's suffering or to restore his spiritual health than visiting with his sister.

Later I spoke to the medical student Philip to thank him for his efforts. I learned that he was a graduate of Notre Dame's School of Global Affairs and Peace Studies under the tutelage of the dean, Dr. Scott Appleby, and that Philip's education there had motivated his kindness. Dean Appleby was one of my mom's favorite high school students and had starred in her Shakespeare plays. I was heartened to see a thread that ran all the way back to my living room on Mockingbird Lane in Shreveport so many years earlier.

I felt proud that Vanderbilt was one of the first hospitals to reopen family visitation during the COVID-19 pandemic, as I knew how powerful the benefits of family and loved ones were for patients—and all of us health-care workers—especially during dying. I had witnessed some devastating scenes in the early months when family were denied access to patients, and I was aware that many people across the world were still unable to be with loved ones just when they were needed the most. This resurgence of antiquated visiting restrictions, not seen in most US ICUs since the 1990s, was traumatizing to patients, family, and health-care workers alike. I read reports on death certificates stating, "Cause of Death: New onset heart failure due to social isolation." One actually said, "Malignant Loneliness." In her thoughtful and urgent book *Elderhood*, geriatrician Dr. Louise Aronson highlights the negative effects of loneliness on well-being, especially among older people, and cites a paper that proves the impact of social isolation on our health is equivalent to smoking fifteen cigarettes a day. When all else is medically equal, loneliness increases mortality by 26 percent. We should be doing everything we can to bring family and friends to our patients both in and out of the hospital.

It is important to stop treating family as visitors to the ICU and to include them as part of the care team, as essential workers, especially during unprecedented times. They are not a luxury but are part of the treatment plan. In addition, we must acknowledge the anxiety that accompanies critical illness for family, and the stress that sometimes increases as a patient's care moves away from cure and into comfort. As they manage their own lives, jobs, children, they are called on to make complicated and painful decisions about their loved ones—all while grieving with the prospect of loss. They must be better informed in making these choices and better supported in carrying them out. They need our respect, our time, and our attention.

• • •

When Mrs. Susan Keener contracted coronavirus, she progressed rapidly to ARDS and needed both mechanical ventilation and ECMO to keep her alive and to give her damaged lungs time to mend. I assumed her care three weeks later. She had partially recovered, but then she developed blockages in the main arteries of both her legs below the knees. Her feet became like blocks of ice, swollen with blood and fluid, the skin on her soles shedding in sheets. It was gruesome to behold. She stayed like this for two to three days, too ill to tolerate amputation, just shy of dying. Her daughter Autumn told me, as we stood together at the bedside, that her mother worked with special needs children and kept in touch with her students even decades later.

Autumn, thirty-five years old and the mother of four young children, was serving as surrogate decision maker. She struggled and cried during our difficult family conference. Her mother was only fifty-three years old. This was so unexpected. I needed to understand better Mrs. Keener's preferences to avoid a potentially catastrophic code blue. "My mom is my best friend," Autumn sobbed. "We've never even had a real fight. She's the absolute best mom anyone could ever have. I just don't know what I'm going to do." I sat with the family, helping them navigate their way forward in this impossible situation. A little while later, Mrs. Keener accidentally removed her breathing tube and looked so peaceful without it that the family and team elected to let her life take its natural course without her going back on the ventilator.

Remarkably, though, instead of dying, she rallied. Her vasopressor needs went from high doses of medication to just a whiff. Her dialysis began working much better, and by the next morning she was on just six liters of oxygen with saturations above 94 percent. Her feet took on color and became much warmer. Soon she was able to sit up in bed, look at pictures of her family trip to Disney World, listen to her favorite Garth Brooks songs, and talk to her family. To love and be loved. This reprieve lasted seventy-two hours. Then the shock returned, and she died with her family at her side, in peace. While the temptation may have been to turn toward devastation, Autumn said instead, "What a gift this time was. I'll have that always."

For me, the entire experience had a certain holiness, one that I often sense in the ICU. It transcends creed or religion and seems to wait in the wings, there when we pause for a moment and take the time to listen.

• • •

When I was a boy, I stumbled upon a dented metal tube in an antique store while shopping with my mom. Nothing special, until the owner suggested I look inside and give it a twist. I peered in awe at a world of ever-changing shapes and color. A kaleidoscope. Since then I have always kept one with me, and sometimes when I have a moment between patients, I dive deep into its world. For me, it is an antidote to burnout. A reminder to go beyond the surface of diagnoses and test results, and machines into the remarkable, colorful, and ever-changing lives of my patients. To find out who they are, and share in all life's messiness. There I find my meaning and purpose as a doctor, as a human. The kaleidoscope is especially helpful as my patients are dying.

In October 2019, a report released by the National Academy of Medicine found that as many as half of the country's doctors and nurses experience substantial symptoms of burnout (and this was before the COVID-19 pandemic), resulting in an increased risk to patients, malpractice claims, worker absenteeism, suicide, and depression, as well as billions of dollars in losses to the medical industry each year. Burnout is a loss of morale felt when people sense their vocation is at odds with their life, rather than harmoniously entwined. Many health-care workers are exhausted, have lost their sense of personal pride or achievement in clinical care, and have become depleted of empathy. This professional crisis has many causes, including long work hours, disaffection with computerization, tedium related to assigning correct codes to diagnoses and procedures, and numerous time constraints that impede patient contact. Add to this our constant exposure to death and the increasingly common feeling that we are missing the personal bedside touch of being doctors, and we have a recipe for personal bankruptcy. To me, the most heartbreaking cause of burnout among health-care professionals is a loss of moral agency combined with an acquisition of learned helplessness, as if we are powerless to change the system.

The National Academy's report made clear that compassionate care is not only better for patients, but also leads to significantly less burnout for doctors and nurses. The 3 Wishes Project proved that nurses who elicited and carried out wishes for their dying patients felt lower levels of distress. For too long, we have been taught to be detached from our patients to spare ourselves emotional pain—"What if your patient dies?"—but the science states that all this does is send our feelings inward, where they churn in negative ways. If, instead, we let ourselves share in our patients' full range of emotions and include the possibility that they may die, then we are better able to care for them—and for ourselves.

Every day, I intentionally try to cultivate compassion and love within the minute-to-minute practice of medicine. This deliberate focus keeps the drift toward burnout at bay. First, as I "foam in and foam out" of each patient's room, I remind myself to approach my patient with empathy. Second, I immediately try to make eye contact and touch the patient to secure human connection, amid the technology of the ICU. When delirium or coma impairs interaction, it drives me to enforce A2F bundle concepts to restore consciousness as soon as possible. Rarely have I told anyone what I'm doing as I pursue these steps as an ICU physician, yet they are vital to my practice of caring for patients. They keep me coming back for more.

In a *JAMA* paper, Dr. Donna Zulman and author-physician Dr. Abraham Verghese, both of Stanford University, identified five ways to help doctors connect with their patients and find meaning for themselves: prepare with intention; listen intently and completely; agree on what matters most; connect with the patient's story; explore emotional cues. For my sickest patients, those who have stopped being able to eat,

I offer a touch of honey on a spoon. They can't aspirate on it, it tastes sweet, and it's a simple gesture of care and affection from one human to another. So much compassion in one small action.

As Drs. Stephen Trzeciak and Anthony Mazzarelli state in their thought-provoking book, *Compassionomics*, "Compassion matters . . . in not only meaningful but measurable ways." It can save patients, families, and the entire crew. They discovered that it takes less than sixty seconds for a physician to make a compassionate connection with a patient and can be accomplished by beginning with a simple statement: "What you're going through is difficult, and I am going to stay with you and not leave you." Compassion is a skill, not a trait, meaning that it can be taught. To be successful, students must want to change and believe that they can change. For me, the most important point made by Drs. Trzeciak and Mazzarelli is that the best doctoring combines technical expertise and compassion.

In my end-of-life conversations, while always remaining kind, I avoid providing false hope. I was once explaining to a daughter that her mother was dying on the ventilator, a conclusion I had come to over five days as, despite everything we had done, no reprieve was in sight from her progressive organ dysfunction. The once-placid daughter slammed her fist on the table, then raised it at me as I recoiled. She stormed out, and I finished the conversation with her sister. A surprised yet inquisitive medical student asked me how I remained poised and hadn't appeared agitated. I told her I believed the daughter had reached a personal ceiling of grief and was not acting like herself due to the immense stress. Moments later, when I went into the room to sit with her at her mother's bedside, we unpacked what had happened. I asked what her mom would want at this stage. She said her mom loved poetry, so we started with Emily Dickinson: "'Hope' is the thing with feathers - That perches in the soul - And sings the tune without the words - And never stops - at all -." There was hope even in the face of death. It was a restorative moment for all of us.

• • •

Studies in the medical literature show that about three out of four hospitalized patients prefer that their physicians ask about and address their spirituality. Most broadly defined, spirituality is the way one experiences, expresses, and/or seeks meaning and purpose. I try to take a "spiritual history" to demonstrate respect for each patient's path, whatever it might be. I usually say, "Do you have any spiritual values that you would like us to know about?" In response, I have heard a huge variety of answers. Never have I had a patient express resistance to or indignation at the question. Another approach I take is to ask, "You are going through something very difficult today, and I'd like to help you as much as possible, so can you tell me a bit about how you deal with stress in your life?" Then I follow my patient's lead or the one provided by loved ones.

Asking a patient who is facing a potentially life-ending illness about her spirituality is broad in that it allows her to opine about her approach to transcendence, yet it is also narrow because of the inherent individuality she brings to the topic. I wholeheartedly embrace getting an answer such as "Thanks for asking. I'm an atheist and don't want any discussion of God or life after death." My answer to him would be "Absolutely, this is why I asked, and I'm going to make sure our team is aware of your preferences."

My team and I have helped to facilitate meditation and prayer services in many of our patients' rooms as they near death. We have brought in prayer rugs and tasbih beads for our Muslim patients and families, allowing them to fulfill their five daily prayers during their last days. We have enabled Hindu family members to set up a small shrine to Ganesh or other gods, and we have also arranged for a Hindu priest to come pray with them. For our Jewish families, we have lit Shabbat candles (far away from the ventilator) and watched over them, letting them flicker briefly, a gesture, before we need to snuff them safely out. All these activities are driven by the patients and their families.

Shortly after one of my patients told me she was an atheist and didn't believe in an afterlife, I witnessed a powerful end-of-life event between her and her family. An esteemed scientist, she asked each of her family members three times, the cadence slightly different each time, "Do you love me?" They affirmed, "Yes," and she gave them a hug and a kiss. Then she asked twice more, followed each time by another hug and kiss, no small feat of courage because she had intense pain from metastatic cancer and a fresh abdominal surgical incision. The emotion was raw, each family member open and exposed. They seemed to move beyond quick answers to thinking about the depth of their love, what it meant to them. To her. She had asked not to be knocked out with morphine, wanting to be present for her loved ones. In completing her ritual, she turned to her other doctor and me and said, "You are part of my inner circle now," then reached out to grant us the same enduring gift. We were stunned by her generosity and felt wholly unworthy.

Dr. Paisal Jirut, a surgeon in the Thai Royal Navy and veteran physician who practiced physical medicine and rehabilitation, answered my questions about his spiritual needs by writing on his whiteboard, "I am meditating each day, but need monks from my temples, please." Immediately we saw to his wish by calling the temples and working with the family. He died surrounded by his three children and his wife, while three Thai Buddhist monks, draped in orange robes that symbolize the flame of truth, chanted prayers into the ether.

When I diagnosed navy veteran Mike Melton with spinocerebellar ataxia, a progressive degenerative disease like ALS, he wanted to figure out a way to marry his girlfriend, Jamie, the love of his life whom he had met on a cycling trip. Mike built bikes for US cyclist and Tour de France winner Greg LeMond and the US Olympic cycling team, pioneering the use of carbon in the industry. He always sported a red, white, and blue bandanna, even with a hospital gown. A few calls and several hours later, a priest was standing at Mike's bedside in the ICU. Our team had decorated the room with white flowers and ribbons, and soft music played. Jamie, all smiles in a flowing green dress, stood next to Mike, who removed his bandanna, and they received the sacrament of matrimony. Their young son, Zachary, clambered up into the bed and laid his head on his father's chest. Later, Jamie told me, "We both had some resentment about not getting married earlier." She took a deep breath. "But this ended up being the perfect timing."

• • •

Several people I love, who are now deceased, suffered from chemical and behavioral addictions, and these experiences affected me deeply. As a student, I struggled with alcohol in a way that was harmful to others and myself. I am a regular attendee of Al-Anon, a spiritual but nonreligious program that helps family members of people with addiction disorders achieve recovery for themselves and find peace of mind. I treasure all that I have learned through Al-Anon about the many ways some people incorporate a higher power into their daily lives. The twelve steps have brought me a sense of serenity in being small, while meditation throughout the day helps me visualize the bigger picture. I have shed the feeling of responsibility and control of other people's lives, and instead my goal is to meet people where they are, which is always a privilege. When Cardinal Ratzinger, who later became Pope Benedict XVI, was asked how many paths there are to God, his answer was "As many paths as there are people." As a practicing Catholic, this to me is a perfect answer, embracing the literal definition of the word *catholic*, which means "universal."

One day, a colleague who became a patient experienced his own need to surrender to his higher power and made a request that touched me profoundly. Dr. Giancarlo Piano, a sixty-four-year-old vascular surgeon in previously perfect physical condition, contracted COVID-19. His wife of thirty-eight years, Mariann, a professor of nursing at Vanderbilt, told me she was scared. Even though his oxygen saturations were holding in the nineties, she said, "He's just too short of breath." Within a week, Giancarlo was admitted to our COVID-ICU, huffing on a BiPAP mask to help with his labored breathing caused by the double pneumonia evident on his chest CT scan. We ramped up his medical care, and I took his spiritual history. "I'm Catholic," he said, taking in a shallow, rattly breath. "Could I receive the Eucharist?"

As a lay minister in the Catholic Church, I can give Communion, offering the Eucharist in the form of sacramental bread and wine, which we believe is transformed into Christ's body and blood during the Mass. The next morning, I went to Mass, then to Giancarlo's room. He was sitting in a chair near the window wearing a high-flow nasal oxygen cannula. After a gentle hello and a glance at his monitor, I knelt in front of him and pulled out a pyx, a small vessel used to carry the Eucharist to Catholics unable to receive it in church. We made the sign of the cross together, and I said, "Gian, from the Holy Gospel according to John, after the miracle of the loaves and fishes, 'Do not labor for food that perishes, but for that which endures unto life everlasting, which the Son of Man will give you.'"

As he consumed the Eucharist, Giancarlo began to sob. I was startled by the emotional intensity and watched as his pulse and breathing skyrocketed. "Breathe, Giancarlo. Please breathe!" I implored him, concerned he might go into cardiac arrest. He began to settle down, and I wiped tears from his cheeks. "You have no idea how much this means to me," he said. "This is the most important thing I could ever want. This is my golden wish."

As physicians, Gian and I incorporate science into our faith, acknowledging that when we ingest the Eucharist, it enters the workings of the cells in our body. My faith affirms that consuming the Eucharist helps me become a better servant of God and others (and I readily admit that I need all the help I can get). I believe that how we handle ourselves on earth will echo into eternity, and the Eucharist is both our shield of protection during life and our viaticum, food for the journey, in dying.

For Gian, the knowledge that this might be the last time he received the Eucharist transformed the moment for him, transporting him beyond the sterile walls of his ICU to a place where he felt safe, loved, and in an eternal relationship with God.

Dr. Giancarlo Piano, a physician, scientist, husband, father, patient, and a friend, desired to be equipped with what he believed to be the only food that will never perish. I was humbled beyond expression to meet his request. A few weeks later, Giancarlo succumbed to COVID-19, surrounded by his wife and sons. As I reflect on our experience together, I remain grateful for his quest and for its intersection with mine.

• • •

Shonda was a young woman with a huge personality. When I met her, she was in her early twenties, and her extraordinary charisma made it seem as if she were already in the exam room when she was still in the waiting area. Unfortunately, she came to me with hemophagocytic lymphohistiocytosis (HLH), an autoimmune disease in which damaged blood cells start to pack the liver, spleen, and even the brain. After taking samples from her hip, we found that her bone marrow was eating itself, which meant that, even with plans for chemotherapy, she and I were on a near-certain path toward her death. Shonda beamed at me excitedly, saying, "I'm a fighter! Everyone knows it."

People, including me, frequently use the metaphor of battle or war when discussing serious illnesses, especially those treated in the ICU. It can be problematic, setting up patients as winners or losers, as if those who care enough about their life and their loved ones persist compared to those who "give up." Equating recovery with strength falsely identifies death and disability with failure and weakness. As with every patient, I knew I would take care of Shonda with all my might. This promise freed me to look after her in the same way whether her illness responded to treatments or whether she continued dying.

Her disease progressed. We gave her more and more red blood cells, platelets, blood pressure medications, chemotherapy, steroids, and antibiotics. Sooner than I expected, though, it became apparent she was not going to make it. The speed of her disease shook me. She was so young, so full of life, but when I sat down with her to tell her, she already knew. It was time to shift the ladder we were climbing from the wall of cure to the wall of comfort. I told her that we would look after her and make her feel safe and heard. We would keep her from suffering and hold her and her loved ones through this time. She was clear in what she wanted: conversations and connection. She hoped to spend time with her young nieces and nephews, and we set up several days of visits in Vanderbilt's sunny hospital courtyard. I watched as they ran here and there, from the shadows back into the light, and she laughed, taking in their joy.

Moment by moment, I tried to approach the sorrow of her dying with an appreciation for spending this time with her. In the past I would have retreated, but this time I plunged in. Her bravery gave me the courage to be vulnerable. To shed my doctor's skin and be wholly human.

As her death grew closer, her loved ones sat by her bedside, still telling stories, still threading their lives to hers. There was love and hope, their sadness bravely held at bay. For her.

Two hours after she had taken her last breath, I was walking by Shonda's room on my way through the busy ICU, where so many lives still hung in the balance. I felt drawn inside and, padding across the floor, I was struck by the silence. The machines were quiet. I peered behind the dividing curtain, expecting the room to be empty. Instead, her figure still lay there on the bed beneath a sheet. I placed a hand on her arm and looked out the large window into the waning sunlight. We had not been doctor and patient, but people. Two humans, small in the big picture. Tears of grief ran down my face, and gratitude, too, for the way she taught me to hold on to the now. I thanked Shonda for the privilege of accompanying her through illness into the beautiful forever.

Epilogue

For every atom belonging to me as good belongs to you.

—Walt Whitman, *Leaves of Grass*

ON A SUNBAKED DAY in the Deep South, I pedaled my squeaky bike to a small library to pull resources for my seventh-grade "research paper"—that's what Mrs. Ilgenfritz called it—answering the question of what I wanted to be when I grew up. In the stacks, I found *Leaves of Grass* and got sidetracked, losing myself in words celebrating the world and the human spirit. I wrote the paper on becoming a physician, but Whitman's poetry is where I found my true answer. I couldn't wait to embark on the exciting adventure of life. With apologies to the Shreveport Memorial Library, I never returned that book.

My journey through critical care is a story about the lives of real people—patients, families, teachers, poets, nurses, and scientists. To me, their lives signify hope. In the years when I lost my way, inchoate and mired in doubt that I might be doing more harm than good, these people brought me back to myself, to the reasons I wanted to become a doctor in the first place. It took me a while to find hope again in critical care, or more specifically to see that hope had always been there. During the often distressing events that I witness every day in the ICU, it can be hard to dispel the power of fear. But I try to remember Nelson Mandela's plea: "May your choices reflect your hopes, not your fears."

In January 2020, I was in a hospital in South Korea for a conference of ICU doctors and nurses, speaking about the vital need to stop sedation as soon as it is safe. During the conference, I examined thirty-two-year-old Yu-hyun Kim, an ICU survivor, who was from the countryside of Gyeonggi Province, just outside Seoul. A couple of years earlier, she had developed diffuse alveolar hemorrhage, a rare disease that caused bleeding into her lungs, and was sedated and immobilized on a ventilator for weeks, leading to a huge loss of her body mass. Now, almost two years after her hospital discharge, she remained frail and in a wheelchair. Her legs were like toothpicks, the muscle on her femurs had wasted away. When I asked why they had sedated her for so long, one of the male intensivists told us, "We were afraid that if we stopped her sedation, she might hurt herself." From across the room, a female colleague countered, "Well, I'm afraid she'll never walk again!"

Over the years, far too many of our decisions in the world of critical care were guided by apprehension. We oversedated patients for too long out of worry that they would experience discomfort and anxiety if we didn't, that they would self-extubate and pull off their restraints. That they would harm us in the throes of delirium-induced violence. We kept patients immobilized due to an overly conservative approach to fall prevention that precluded us from attempting to walk them early. We kept families away from patients, treating loved ones as visitors rather than members of the healing plan, because we thought they would distract us and consume our precious time. We sidestepped conversations about death in the ICU, designating it as a place for saving lives, and we avoided updating our culture of care because it was scary to embrace change. But it was especially frightening to admit that we were wrong in adopting a treatment approach that damaged many people's lives. For me, the only way to right this wrong was to improve the way we care for the world's sickest patients in ICUs.

In the unsettling era of COVID-19, trepidation was again a driver of unparalleled upheaval in the medical community. Doctors and nurses, and all those working in health care, poured everything they had into caring for patients infected with a highly contagious, febrile disease without a cure, one that attacked multiple organs with unrelenting ferocity. Hospital staffers did so with limited personal protective equipment (PPE) in ICUs filled to capacity. Unfortunately, in our rush to respond, we set aside twenty-five years of progress in critical care—outlined in this book—and only loosely applied established protocols for ventilator management and A2F bundle concepts. If mad scientists had schemed to create the greatest number of people with delirium and PICS, COVID-19 and our early response to the pandemic would have been their devious ploy.

In the initial panic, we focused on getting our patients on ventilators, sedating them heavily, and didn't pause to think about downstream effects. We isolated our patients to save our supplies of PPE, stopping early mobility and physical therapy sessions, and we prevented friends and families from visiting. Dr. Robert Hyzy, ICU director at the University of Michigan, told me, "Doctors had a fear of exposing nurses and ourselves to the virus. This drove a willingness to deviate from established practices. Keeping sedation going should immediately trigger fear. But it didn't. That worry was drowned out in our minds by earned fatigue, sore noses from N95s, hunger, and the need to go to the bathroom on a long shift wearing PPE. And the patients don't know about PICS . . . yet."

When I spoke with Dr. Elisabeth Riviello, an ICU doctor at Beth Israel/Harvard in Boston, her words were similar: "The risk of PICS in patients we sedate too heavily and too long is less dramatic, and further away from our thoughts, than the need to save their lives, so we give in to more immediate fears and keep people sedated."

Though we knew better, our ICUs became delirium factories all over again, launching an enduring public health crisis for a new wave of survivors. Early in the pandemic, we studied more than two thousand COVID-ICU patients in fourteen countries, and the science showed that overuse of benzodiazepines and underuse of families at the bedside were contributing to delirium and death. In 1896, Sir William Osler wrote, "Humanity has but three great enemies, fever, famine and war; of these, by far the greatest, by far the most terrible, is fever." The pandemic was fever, and when we added fear to fever, the results were catastrophic.

• • •

My odyssey in medicine started at Charity Hospital in New Orleans in 1985. During the pandemic, I was in daily contact with some of my former pulmonary and critical care fellows, who became attending physicians turned COVID doctors caring for patients in Louisiana. They were slammed with coronavirus cases, half a dozen very sick people showing up at their hospitals every hour or so.

Dr. Hollis "Bud" O'Neal, ICU research director at Our Lady of the Lake hospital in Baton Rouge, provided me with much-needed wisdom as the COVID surge began in Nashville: "We're hearing some physicians recommend radically new approaches to COVID-19. All I know is that deviating from lifesaving methods proven over twenty years will do more harm than good. For my patients, I'm sticking to the A2F bundle. We know it works."

I found his words inspiring in an uncertain world. Eventually, as doctors and nurses found their footing with COVID, learning more about the disease and its impacts on the human body, there was a return to established protocols and best practices, including basic tenets of ventilator management and major elements of the A2F bundle. We found safe ways to release patients from the grip of sedation, move them out of bed earlier, and hold their loved ones again. In the initial stages, we saw only a new disease, one we were determined to eradicate with new treatments, come what may. Later, we saw that we could best handle this virus in ways we already knew, tried-and-true approaches. We turned to our past to ground us and help us find our way in the face of the unknown. My medical school roommate, Dr. Darin Portnoy, a former president of Doctors Without Borders USA, told me, "It was eerily similar during the Ebola crisis. We were blindsided and we scrambled at first, but then we returned to what we already knew."

In *Being Mortal*, Dr. Atul Gawande outlines the stark reality that too often, in modern times, we disregard the wisdom of those who have the most experience. He pointed out that in former generations, so much respect was shown to elders that people pretended to be older rather than younger. Dr. Gawande teaches that "as for the exclusive hold that elders once had on knowledge and wisdom, that, too, has eroded, thanks to technologies of communication. . . . At one time, we might have turned to an old-timer to explain the world. Now we consult Google, and if we have any trouble with the computer, we ask a teenager." In critical care, my elders, often my mentors, remember when we tried nontraditional resuscitation strategies, new medications, and experimental ventilator settings, and how they failed. I turn to my elders not because they are always right, but because of the insights and knowledge they possess from previous mistakes.

I have a practice whereby I actively seek the wisdom of my elderly patients. In taking a patient's history, if I learn that she's been married for fifty years or more, I stop what I'm doing, sit down, and listen to her story. Two couples, both married over sixty years, became my life coaches during COVID. The first was Mrs. Virginia Stevens and Mr. Doyle Thomas "DT" Stevens. Married sixty-six years when the pandemic broke out, both eighty-eight years old and with progressive COVID infections, they were admitted to our unit in rooms down the hall from each other. I found DT exasperated and grappling to get out of his bed, insisting, "I have to find Virginia. Where did they take her?" It was the only thing he could think about. The nurses said he was belligerent with delirium all morning, that he was unable to eat until they tried a touch of honey on a spoon. For hope and healing. For a few minutes, his brain cleared, and he calmed down. But then he sought Virginia again. Through some stellar work by the Stevenses' attending physician and the nursing staff, we were able to transfer him into her room. What a difference that made. His delirium quickly receded. I cherish the picture I have of us together, me in my yellow PPE and N95, and them, mattress to mattress, gripping each other's hands as if they will never let go again, smiling in recovery. On discharge, their daughter, Karen, echoed what I was thinking: "We had the most kind, helpful, compassionate, respectful nurses I've ever seen. Beyond exceptional." Many months into the pandemic and exhausted beyond words, the nurses had exceeded themselves. As usual, they all assured me they received from Mr. and Mrs. Stevens much more than they gave. Again, I thought, "*Cada persona es un mundo.*" "Each person is a world."

Just a few weeks later, Mary and Phillip Hill, married sixty-one years, both developed fever and shortness of breath. Due to delays and conflicting test results, they spent days being cared for by their children, Kathy, Gigi, and David. Eventually both parents and their daughters were diagnosed with COVID, but only Mary and Phillip were sick enough to require hospitalization. Phillip had previously received a heart transplant and was immunosuppressed, and as his was a potentially complex case, he was moved two hours east to our COVID-ICU, while Mary remained at the local hospital. For days, the family tried to get her transferred, and as both Mary's and Phillip's condition worsened with no expectation of recovery, the family made impassioned pleas. Kathy said, "I live my life to minimize regrets, and I told Mom's doctor that if they were going to die, I had to get them together." The physician didn't seem to understand the urgency, stating that the transfer would not change Mary's outcome, so there would be no point medically, and beds were scarce. At Vanderbilt, however, Phillip's physicians disagreed. They made sure the room next to Phillip's remained open for his wife, to ensure these two soul mates could be together.

Kathy said, "A few days later I called Daddy to tell him that Momma was being transferred, and they would be in adjacent rooms with the same care, the same nurses, the same doctors. Together." After five long days of being apart, Mary and Phillip saw each other once again. At first, they were separated by a wall, but their nursing team dreamed bigger and set Mary up for all her medical care in Phillip's room. Now they lay next to each other with thick, corrugated high-flow oxygen tubing whooshing air into their bodies. Mary looked over at her husband, her hand reaching out to touch his wrist, bruised from blood draws, as she repeated, "Phil, I'm here. I'm here." They were together again. Three weeks into their struggle with COVID, ten days after their initial hospitalization, and two days after their nurses placed them in the same room, they died within a few hours of each other, holding hands and surrounded by family. Kathy told me, "We never left the room. The nurses took care of us all day—fed us box lunches and brought us a basket of snacks. They were beyond kind."

Even amid the fear, hope flared.

Seeing the Stevenses and the Hills, the couples steadfast in their love for each other after so much time, made me reflect on my own marriage and family. Our children are grown now, have graduated from college, and are pursuing vocations of their own. Kim and I, over thirty years into marriage, have more time for each other and are deepening our relationship and relishing its maturity. I am reminded of advice given by theologian and anti-fascist Dietrich Bonhoeffer in a letter he wrote to his niece from a Nazi prison camp: "It is not your love that sustains the marriage, but from now on, the marriage that sustains your love." It prompts me to think of my role as a doctor, too, and how it's bigger than just me caring for my patients. The relationship is reciprocal, and my patients provide inspiration and meaning to sustain me.

• • •

I remember well the first day I met Clementine Hunter. I was nine years old, and my uncle Warren and I had started early that morning, rumbling down the road in his Datsun pickup. A new mattress, wrapped in my grandma's homemade quilts, bounced around in the back. Uncle Warren collected art, encountering little-known artists by word of mouth or by seeing their works propped up outside their homes. Clementine was the first artist he had brought me to visit, and we were taking her supplies. I rode next to him, paints, brushes, and canvas on my left, my arm draped out the window on the right. It's hot in Louisiana, and morning was the rare time of day when I felt cool air blowing on my face. I breathed it in, riding beside my uncle, bounding down tar roads from Shreveport to Melrose Plantation, where Clementine lived.

Uncle Warren turned down a dusty driveway and stopped in front of a small shotgun house, its white paint chipped and weathered by the relentless Southern sun. Clementine was there, sitting on the front porch, just like every screen porch I ever saw, with rips in the old metal screen. Bent over and smiling, she swung the door open, making its rusted hinges squeak. She must have been in her eighties. "How y'all doin'?" she asked, welcoming us.

An easel was on the porch, and another was just inside the front room. Red, green, yellow, and white oil paint was smeared across her worn hands, and I could see a painting she was working on, a baptismal procession with Black women dressed all in white, strolling from a hilltop church toward the pond below, where a full-dunk baptism was taking place. Uncle Warren had told me she was a memory painter, transferring scenes in her mind onto the canvas. Seeing me looking, she leaned in and hugged me and led me inside to the other easel, with the beginnings of a new painting.

"This one of the honky-tonk'll be for you, Wes," she said. "I call it *Saturday Night*." I leaned in and watched her paint, thick brushstrokes of bright color. As she worked, she told me that life is hard, that people fight and suffer, but they dance, too. The painting would remind me of that. "You'll have to make up your mind what you're gonna do more, fight or dance."

Epilogue

Later, Uncle Warren and I heaved the mattress off the truck and laid it in place in the back room, taking the shoddy old one away. As the evening sky's intense red faded to pink and then into blackness, we headed for home. Clementine waved goodbye from her porch. She had a better night's sleep in store.

When the painting *Saturday Night* was finished, Uncle Warren bought it for me, and it now hangs in my house, a memorial of that day and all the other days I spent with Uncle Warren and Clementine. We often took her paints and brushes, sometimes homemade red beans and rice with spicy Cajun sausage, small things to make her life easier. Now I know that her ancestors were slaves who had worked at Melrose, picking cotton from morning until night, and that Clementine herself had once worked in the fields, then as a housemaid and cook. I had seen the two-story house with its white columns across the street, the brick walk curving under an oak tree draped in Spanish moss. Clementine received no formal education and never had the chance to learn to read or write. But one day in the 1940s, some guests who were artists had left their paints in a drawer. As she cleaned up, rather than throw them away, something drew her to scavenge a discarded cloth window shade from the trash and paint a scene from her memory.

That started a habit, a calling, and she created one painting after another depicting life, often many paintings of the same theme—picking cotton, weddings, funerals, Saturday night, going to church—until she died at the age of 101. She became one of the most famous of all Southern folk artists, and was even invited to the White House. Her work has been displayed at famous galleries such as the Louvre in Paris, the American Folk Art Museum in New York, and the Oprah Winfrey Collection in Chicago.

Clementine was treated as "other" throughout her early life, dismissed as poor and inconsequential, depersonalized, until her paintings were discovered. But for me her story is one of light in the darkness. In my mind, she is always standing on her porch, painting, following her calling. She taught me there may be pain and violence in life, and that I could go out in the world and help create more hope and healing.

• • •

A few years ago, I was in Zambia studying delirium along with our global health community partners and Dr. Kondwelani Mateyo, one of the few trained pulmonologists in the country. Zambia struggles, as does much of Africa, with an ongoing HIV/AIDS epidemic, and more than 50 percent of the critically ill patients enrolled in our study were living with HIV. Though this disease can lead to systemic infections that often result in sepsis, and predisposes patients to delirium, there was little evidence available on the subject in Zambia or in other settings with limited resources. As I stood at the bedside of a disoriented woman in an overcrowded ICU, I was reminded of my days at Charity and the rich brew of humanity there that I had so loved. As if reading my mind, Dr. Mateyo looked up and asked, "How is it that a boy from Louisiana ended up here with me in Lusaka?"

I pondered the question throughout the trip. Later as I strolled in a fruit-tree grove that doubled as a cemetery, I saw tombstones draped with flowers and two bright blue and yellow huts where people gave thanks for the lives of their lost loved ones. It was a place of hope. Of gratitude. And yet I knew that many of the dead had succumbed to diseases that could have been treated if they had lived in a country with more resources.

Coming to Zambia was a natural extension of the scientific process of improving medicine that I had been pursuing over the past twenty-five years. I still had the desire to keep my lens focused outward, to help those without a voice. The science of the A2F bundle is proven to save lives and help survivors, and as teams implement new ways in a wider world, we will adapt to meet the needs of each patient population. In countries like Zambia, we are just starting out. There is an element of excitement in that, as change ripples from one ICU to the next. I am confident that doctors like Dr. Mateyo and other leaders in low- and middle-income countries will spread the word across sub-Saharan Africa and beyond, bettering the lives of millions of patients there.

• • •

Recently I spoke with Carla Davis, who leads Heart of Hospice, an organization that provides hospice services for people at the end of life. I was deeply impressed by her compassion and resourcefulness, especially during the pandemic. For her and her team, COVID ignited a need to serve every dying patient they could, many of whom were refused care from other hospice agencies, which felt ill-equipped to help them.

Without question Heart of Hospice was going to do everything it could to get involved. "Once we sourced PPE, we recruited about eighty nervous but willing staff from three states to fill all the slots in Louisiana," Carla said. "The early surge was so abysmal." Within the first few months, they cared for over 450 dying COVID patients in their homes, even those in shock and on adrenaline drips, who are not usually discharged to hospice as their care is complicated. But a lot of patients were also dying in hospitals, alone and isolated, and didn't have a home to go to.

Undeterred, Carla looked for a suitable place to set up an inpatient center for these patients and found a ventilator facility in New Orleans that had shut down the week before. "From conception to receiving approvals, we took a yearlong process and in ten days had patients in every room." I wondered how they overcame so many obstacles so quickly. "We ran the lanes." I could hear the excitement in Carla's voice. "It can't always be linear. It was bam, bam, bam, and as the barriers fell, our dream of serving these people came true like a flash of lightning." When I asked her for one word that encapsulated the entire story, I thought she might say "Chaos." Or "Miracle." Instead she said, "Figs."

She brushed her sandy-blond hair back and smiled. "I was there with my first patient, and I asked her what she wanted us to do for her. In a thick Cajun accent, she said, 'Figs, ya know, they're sweet.'" Someone went out and found her a bunch of purple and gold figs—plump, juicy, and fresh—the kind we love so much in Louisiana. The patient ate every single one before she died three days later.

• • •

As I headed into the unit, I received a text from Tisha Holt: "Thanks for the uplifting message, Dr. Ely. Good wishes like this are getting me through." I smiled. It seemed like such an ordinary moment, a simple response to a text I'd sent earlier in the day. But Tisha was one of the patients I would be rounding on that morning, in the ICU with COVID-19 pneumonia and ARDS. Her lung disease was so severe and her oxygen so low that she was on a ventilator. Without it she would have died. She described the feeling of breathing in and out as like being tangled in barbed wire. Today she was sitting up in bed, propped against the pillows, texting all her friends to tell them she was alive. We had used just enough sedation to "keep the chill off," as she put it, and that afternoon we would be getting her out of bed. Next, we would clothe her parents in PPE and bring them into her room. We were back on track. One patient at a time, one person at a time.

Not so long ago, a friend sent me a video of a spider spinning a web on the porch of his house by the lake. I watched, mesmerized, as it wove intricate threads, circling out from the center to create layer upon layer of a breathtaking structure. I had never seen such an enormous web. Moments later, it seemed, a torrent of rain ripped down the web, sending the spider hurrying for shelter. I felt saddened by the destruction as I watched the spider tiptoe out, sure that it would feel downcast at the loss of its work. Instead it just began weaving again, patiently starting over.

I realized that this was exactly what I needed to do. As the pandemic roared around us, we had to begin again, to keep working on getting our message out, and passing it along from one ICU to the next and the next and down the line, to ensure that the tides of critical care fully shift toward compassionate, safe, and evidence-based care for every patient. My job is to see my patients and all that makes them who they are and continue to care for them to the best of my ability—to save their lives if possible, to prevent them from developing PICS as far as I can, and to support them in their post-ICU survivorship.

If someone had asked me when I was a young doctor about the most important aspects of critical care, I would eagerly have talked about ventilators and vasopressors, and moving patients out of shock and onto life support. I would never have imagined that one day I might answer figs, or honey on a spoon, or a bar of music.

In response to despair, I will do what I always do. I will lean toward hope.

• • •

It seems fitting to close with a story of gratitude and promise. A moment of grace for me and a look to the future, too. For several years now, I have tried to trace Teresa Martin, to find the young woman whose life I tried so hard to save over thirty years ago, only to send her home alive, for sure, but with new brain and body diseases. With PICS. When I finally tracked down her medical file, I learned that she had died not so long ago, but I connected with her grown-up son, Travis Martin. I told him how sorry I was about his mother, about the damage I had done. I realized that he was there the night she overdosed and landed in the ICU, that he was the reason she regretted her actions and was determined to live.

Travis didn't have much of a childhood, helping his mother in and out of her wheelchair and filling in for her when her memory gave out. He didn't know it, but he had suffered his entire life with PICS-F, struggling with depression and PTSD. I thought he might be angry about what happened to his mom, but he wasn't. He had found his way to therapy, his own downstream solution, and it had helped him to gain peace. When I explained, one more time, that I had been trying to save his mother's life, and that I have spent the rest of my life striving to help other patients navigate critical illness, he stopped me:

"You know, I've been working on my wife's car, and there's a certain way that things are done. It may have been done differently ten, twenty years ago, but somewhere somebody improved it. It sounds like you've identified something similar. We constantly need to improve medicine to help people is what you're trying to say."

I nodded, a lump in my throat. He was exactly right. It's what I've been trying to say and do all this time.

Resources for Patients, Families, Caregivers, and Medical Professionals

AS I CONSIDERED THE best way to present practical tips for readers, torrents of rain pounded on the tin roof of the mountain cabin I was visiting. I heard branches breaking, and thunder clapped overhead. In the middle of such a treacherous storm, my safety felt tenuous. It made me think of other precarious times in my life, and I pondered your future need of refuge from a squall. In times of crisis, this is all we really want: shelter from the storm.

I hope that in addition to the stories and truths in *Every Deep-Drawn Breath*, these resources offer you a path forward amid the uncertainty and vulnerability of life during and following critical illness. The Critical Illness, Brain Dysfunction, and Survivorship (CIBS) Center posts all our resources free of charge at www.icu delirium.org. We are an independently run, non-industry-funded educational resource, and we invite you to browse our website for more information.

Each person's illness and recovery path is unique. As such, there is no substitute for talking directly with your doctor, nurse, pharmacist, occupational and physical therapist, rehabilitation specialist, social worker, spiritual adviser or chaplain, and other members of your health-care team. The information that follows is secondary and supplementary to those conversations.

In creating these resources, Dr. Caroline Lassen-Greene and Dr. James C. Jackson, who run our ICU support groups as psychologists in the CIBS Center, provided helpful insights. Additional thanks go to the many dedicated teams who crafted educational materials found on websites listed at the end of this section.

This section addresses the following topics:

- Understanding Delirium: A Guide for Loved Ones during Hospitalization and Beyond
- Tips for Dealing with Delirium
- Resources for Medical Team Members
- A General Guide to PICS for Patients and Families
- After the ICU—A PICS Survivor's Guide from the Patient's Perspective
- Debunking Myths about the Aging Brain
- Boosting Your Brain Health
- Helpful Websites

UNDERSTANDING DELIRIUM: A GUIDE FOR LOVED ONES DURING HOSPITALIZATION AND BEYOND

When you go to the hospital, you or your loved one might end up with delirium: a sudden change in thinking and behavior manifested primarily as an inability to pay attention or follow commands. It could start with you asking, "Am I getting confused? Is he or she confused?" It may seem odd, but patients often do have the capacity to realize when they are getting confused. Delirium can affect people at any age, but older patients in the hospital and especially in the ICU are at highest risk. About two out of three patients in the ICU develop delirium, and many patients suffer from delirium while they are on a breathing machine or soon afterward. Delirium may begin rapidly or come on gradually; it may emerge and depart quickly or last for days to weeks. Delirium is a dangerous condition that represents a global problem with the way a person's brain is working and is a risk factor for a higher likelihood of death, longer length of stay in the hospital, higher cost of care, and the development of thinking and memory problems that can last for months and even years. It is extremely important that you are aware of the potential for your loved one to develop delirium during a hospital stay and to be on the lookout for it.

Patients may:

- Be confused
- Have attention and memory problems
- Be unable to focus or follow directions
- Seem as if they are "not themselves"
- Appear agitated or, alternatively, uncharacteristically quiet
- Be aggressive
- Have drastic emotional changes
- Be unsure about where they are
- Be unsure about the time of day
- Act differently from usual
- Use inappropriate words that are out of character for them
- See things that are not there
- Have changes in sleeping habits
- Have movements that are not typical for them, such as tremors or picking at clothes

Delirium is caused by a change in the way the brain is working. This can be brought on or made worse by:

- Less oxygen to the brain
- Chemical changes in the brain
- Certain medications
- Infections
- Severe pain
- Medical illnesses (preexisting and current)
- Unfamiliar surroundings
- Alcohol, sedatives, or painkillers
- Withdrawal from nicotine, alcohol, narcotics, or sedatives

People most likely to develop delirium are those who:

- Have dementia or even mild cognitive problems
- Are advanced in age
- Have had surgery, especially hip or heart
- Have depression or other preexisting psychiatric conditions
- Take certain high-risk medicines
- Have poor eyesight or hearing
- Have an infection or sepsis
- Have heart failure

The next section addresses what you should do if you think that your loved one is at risk to develop delirium or suspect she has delirium.

TIPS FOR DEALING WITH DELIRIUM

If you or a family member is facing hospitalization or surgery, take steps to help prevent or reduce the duration of delirium.

Preparation for Hospitalization

- "Prehab" for any planned surgeries or hospitalizations: prepare as if you were training for a sports event (exercise, eat a healthy diet, and get good sleep).
- Bring a list of your current medications and supplements.
- Ask for delirium/cognitive screening before and after elective surgeries.
- Bring hearing aids, eyeglasses, and dentures and use them.
- Ask a friend or family member to stay with you 24-7 if allowed.

During Hospitalization

- Whenever possible, get exposure to sunlight during the day and only remain in the bed when required.
- Mobilize early and often. Walk as soon as possible after the procedure.
- Remember that natural sleep following fatigue from exercise is much better than medication-induced sleep or sedation.

- Close the door to your room, use earplugs and a sleep mask, or bring a familiar pillow or blanket to sleep better. And, yes, these are options in the ICU for many patients.

For Caregivers (loved ones and even health-care professionals)

- Seek medical help if you notice your loved one is "just not him- or herself."

- Validate your loved one's suffering and give reassurance that measures are being taken to ensure comfort. This step reminds you to maintain your loved one's dignity and humanity.

- Communicate with the health-care team and ask if any active medications your loved one is on will increase the risk of delirium.

- Ensure that pain is adequately controlled (often family will know better than the team).

- Ask for a consult with a psychiatrist, neurologist, or geriatrician (for older patients) if you have lingering questions.

- If your loved one develops delirium, provide verbal orientation and reassurance.

- Reintroduce yourself and members of the health-care team.

- Explain to your loved one the specific plan for the day.

- Be patient with your loved one. Speak gently, repeat yourself often, and use simple words or phrases.

- Remind the patient of the day, date, and situation—
  orient the patient as much and as often as possible by
  talking about current events in your life and in the
  news.

- Talk about family, friends, and familiar topics.

- Decorate the room with calendars or family
  pictures. These familiar items might be reminders
  of home and provide hope at a key time.

- Talk with the medical team about the best way to
  provide the patient with his or her favorite music or,
  when awake, TV shows.

- Ask your nurse for an ICU diary and start to build a
  personal record of your loved one's hospital stay with
  notes, photos, and videos. Chronicling details of
  each day can be helpful later in putting the pieces of
  the stay back together.

- Work with the medical team to help your loved
  one safely get out of bed and moving as soon as
  possible.

- Make sure your loved one has glasses, hearing aids,
  and dentures as needed.

- Play simple games such as tic-tac-toe, word jumble,
  crossword puzzles, and sudoku with your loved one
  to keep his or her brain active.

- Prepare to assist cognitively after leaving the hospital
  because brain fog can last a long time.

Sensory Improvement

If applicable, ensure the patient has:

- Hearing aid batteries
- Eyeglass wipes
- Reading glasses
- Magnifier
- Denture adhesive and cleaner
- List of medications

For sleep promotion

- Safe, monitored mobilization to generate fatigue
- Eye mask
- Earplugs
- Relaxation via a special TV channel, music, or audiobooks

When appropriate, try to engage the patient with the following:

- Puzzles
- Crayons
- Coloring books
- Playing cards
- Large-print word search or crossword puzzle
- Stuffed animal
- Whatever else you know she or he loves

RESOURCES FOR MEDICAL TEAM MEMBERS

The ABCDEF Bundle

The Society of Critical Care Medicine (SCCM) is the backbone behind the ABCDEF (A2F) bundle, an evidence-based safety bundle developed between 2005 and 2020 and the foundation of the SCCM's ICU Liberation Collaborative (www.icudelirium.org and www.iculib eration.org). This movement was an outgrowth of the patients' stories told in this book, which led physician-scientists and their research teams the world over to design landmark cohort studies and clinical trials that revealed startling improvements in care now encapsulated in the A2F bundle. This has been a global effort contributed to by countless people, funding agencies, and, most important, patients and families.

Here is an outline of the six components of the A2F bundle:

- **A**nalgesia: assess, prevent, manage pain
- **B**oth SATs and SBTs: stop drugs, stop ventilator
- **C**hoice of analgesia and sedation
- **D**elirium: assess, prevent, manage
- **E**arly mobility and exercise, environment
- **F**amily engagement and empowerment

The concepts covered in these six safety steps of the A2F bundle are essential to rehumanizing our patients amid the technologically driven ICU environment. They are a means to ensure we avoid the trap of unintended and unwarranted chemical and physical restraints that harm people. Health-care providers can take specific steps to help prevent or lessen the severity of delirium. These steps are often inexpensive and require few resources and little specialized training. Frequently they involve asking good questions and relying on tried-and-true clinical skills.

Evaluate whether your patient is:

- Overmedicated
- Lacking oxygen
- Immobilized unnecessarily
- Dehydrated
- Not warm enough
- Constipated
- Lacking food
- Lacking sleep

Recommendations:

- Warn patients and family members of the many risks of delirium and advise on how to avoid.
- Look for infections or underlying medical conditions that may be causing delirium.
- Try to manage pain with non-opioid analgesics if possible or the smallest successful doses of opioids.
- Manage delirium using nonpharmacological methods first, such as mobilization and maximizing engagement with loved ones.
- Sedating medications should be avoided whenever possible.
- Do not discharge patients with delirium symptoms unless a competent caregiver is at home.

- Educate others, including caregivers, about delirium and how its emergence following discharge should serve as a warning sign of complications that warrant immediate medical attention.

TIPS FOR ANESTHESIA AND SURGERY

Anesthesiologists can take steps to help prevent and treat delirium:

- *Work as interprofessional teams:* Team members with an array of skill sets optimize care. For example, combine the physician's evaluation with a medication review by a PharmD, delirium screenings before surgery by a nurse, and cognitive "prehab" prior to hospitalization by a psychologist or technician and willing family members.

- *Screen cognitive function:* All patients should be evaluated before surgery for preexisting cognitive decline and delirium risk factors.

- *Reduce deliriogenic medications:* Avoid unnecessary sedatives, anticholinergic medications, and antipsychotics. Instead, look for underlying causes of delirium and utilize family members for support.

- *Assess pain-control options:* Use a multimodal pain management plan incorporating options such as local and regional analgesia where possible and non-narcotic pain medications like acetaminophen or gabapentin to minimize opioids. Avoid benzodiazepines.

- *Educate:* Families and health-care providers need to understand how to prevent and treat delirium.

A GENERAL GUIDE TO PICS FOR PATIENTS AND FAMILIES

Note: This section was adapted with permission from the American Thoracic Society's patient and family education series: S. Kosinski, R. A. Mohammad, M. Pitcher et al., American Journal of Respiratory and Critical Care Medicine 201 (2020): 15–16, www.thoracic.org/patients/patient-resources.

• • •

Post-intensive care syndrome (PICS) is a term that was created by a group of experts focused on the needs of ICU survivors. It refers to a condition that develops when a patient experiences new or worsening impairment in the physical, cognitive, or mental domain after critical illness. These impairments may persist after ICU discharge and in some cases represent a "new normal," or a permanent condition. Almost half of all survivors of critical illness who were in the workforce before ICU admission are out of the workforce a year later. One-quarter of survivors require assistance in activities of daily living a year after admission to a critical care unit, and approximately half of families providing care must make a major adjustment to their lives.

Symptoms of PICS

People who develop PICS can experience any combination of these physical, emotional, and cognitive symptoms. They may be entirely new problems or the worsening of problems that were present before the critical illness.

- Physical symptoms such as weakness, decreased endurance, pain, shortness of breath, and difficulty with movement or exercise.

- Mental health symptoms such as anxiety, panic disorder, impaired mood, major depression, sleep problems, and post-traumatic stress disorder.

- Cognitive problems including processing things slowly and difficulty in attending, concentrating, multitasking, and remembering.

Detecting PICS

A health-care provider may detect symptoms or ask about anxiety, depression, breathlessness, the ability to complete daily tasks (such as bathing), and people's overall quality of life and their day-to-day functioning. Patients can complete assessments to gauge the severity of PICS symptoms including cognitive, mental, and physical health testing. Family members may notice their loved one is having difficulty with their health after hospital discharge and should help set up a doctor's appointment.

Who Gets PICS?

PICS can affect any person who survives a critical illness, even people who were healthy prior to their severe illness and hospital stay. PICS is most common among people who were admitted to an ICU, but many people treated outside the ICU can develop this condition as well. The name refers specially to intensive care, but elements of cognitive dysfunction, depression, and physical disability can certainly emerge for some patients during non-ICU hospitalizations. People who had existing health problems, such as lung disease or muscle disorders, prior to a hospitalization are at higher risk of developing PICS. People with psychiatric illness or cognitive impairment (mild cognitive impairment or dementia) are also more likely to have worsening of their symptoms after an ICU stay. Some types of illnesses and events that may occur in the hospital may also increase the risk of developing PICS. For example, people who have severe infections, acute respiratory distress syndrome, delirium, low oxygen levels, and/or low blood pressure during their illness are more likely to get PICS.

Preventing PICS

Several things can be done during a hospitalization that may reduce the risk of developing PICS:

- If a person needs breathing support, the health-care team will try to minimize time on the mechanical ventilator and use only as much sedating medication as is safe.

- Physical therapy can be started early during an illness even while other intensive medical therapy (e.g., mechanical ventilation) is ongoing.

- Delirium monitoring multiple times per day with formal documentation in the medical record is recommended by numerous international guidelines as part of routine care for every patient while in the ICU.

- Family members and health-care providers can keep a diary of events that happen in the hospital to help patients link memories they have during recovery to the care they received. This has proven beneficial to healing weeks, months, and even years later.

- Have family and friends talk with the patient and bring in music and pictures from home.

- Providers can educate patients and families about problems that may develop after ICU discharge so that if they do occur, patients will not be caught off guard and will understand what is happening to them.

Treating PICS

Treatment for PICS depends on the specific symptoms:

- Several multidisciplinary clinics provide support for patients after critical illness, and primary care physicians should be educated about and involved in this complex care. Treatment plans may involve several professionals working as a team. Psychologists, social workers, pharmacists, physical therapists, occupational therapists, nurses, and physicians may each contribute to the recovery.

- Weakness and deconditioning can be treated with physical therapy and exercise programs.

- Mental health symptoms such as depression, anxiety, or PTSD can be treated with a combination of therapy and medications.

- Patients and their caregivers may find it beneficial to share stories with one another, to give and receive advice. Support groups for ICU survivors are especially helpful.

- If cognitive impairment results in difficulty thinking, remembering, or concentrating, a formal evaluation by a neurocognitive specialist may help, and a plan for cognitive therapy can be developed.

- Occupational therapy may help ICU survivors manage these new difficulties and improve symptoms.

- Helping the patient feel heard and validated and having their symptoms taken seriously are crucial.

How Long Does PICS Last?

PICS symptoms are often present six months to one year after a hospitalization or longer. Every person will have a different recovery. Some symptoms may improve or resolve completely within weeks or months. Unfortunately, in some people, PICS symptoms may last years or even a lifetime. Health-care providers can support people at every stage as they adjust to a new level of functioning after critical illness.

For Caregivers

Critical illness can be difficult for family members and other caregivers. It is too often overlooked that caregivers can experience stress and develop depression, anxiety, or post-traumatic stress disorder even after a loved one is discharged from the hospital. It is important that caregivers find time for self-care, ask for support, and work with their own health-care providers, including professional mental health providers, to manage any symptoms they may have.

PICS and COVID-19

Patients with COVID-19 are at high risk for PICS, which in COVID patients is often called Long COVID or post-acute COVID syndrome (PACS) or post-acute sequelae of SARS-CoV-2 infection (PASC), where *sequelae* refers to a condition that is the result of a previous illness or injury. SARS-CoV-2 is the name of the virus that causes COVID. Patients who suffer ongoing symptoms are referred to as long-haulers. Those who were in the ICU are essentially long-haulers with PICS, an especially egregious form of Long COVID. Some of the reasons PICS is so rampant in ICU survivors after COVID include:

- Constraints on social support while hospitalized

- Prolonged mechanical ventilation

- Exposure to high doses and prolonged use of sedatives (e.g., benzodiazepines)

- Prolonged immobilization and limited physical therapy due to risk of infection transmission and demands outstripping available personnel

- Limited visitation policies resulting in intense isolation from family and friends

- Limited access to post-ICU care due to service limitations and regional restrictions

The way forward through PICS, whether it be after a general ICU stay or as a form of Long COVID, is found in the next section, the PICS survivor's guide.

AFTER THE ICU—A PICS SURVIVOR'S GUIDE FROM THE PATIENT'S PERSPECTIVE

Special thanks to Mr. Audin Huslid, a former ICU patient, who provided foundational material from his survival experience, which he describes as "coming in from the wilderness."

General Remediation

- Educate yourself about PICS and be ready to seek help for yourself if you show any symptoms after discharge.

- Familiarize yourself with your ICU history by reading your medical records and talking to anyone who saw you during that period (e.g., family and friends, nurses, doctors, caseworkers, spiritual advisers, or chaplains).

- Ask to see your ICU diary if one was created during your stay and go through it with a family member who saw you in the hospital.

- If you had delirium in the ICU, realize that the hallucinations you experienced are common. These hallucinations can be distressing, vivid, and involve a range of themes and images including torture, death, or sex. They can return after you have left the ICU.

- Be aware that loved ones of ICU patients may suffer PICS symptoms (typically referred to as PICS-family or PICS-F) from the stress of their own experience in the ICU at the bedside. They also may need to speak with a psychologist or psychiatrist.

Establish Continuity of Care Between the ICU and Post-ICU Doctors and Therapists

- ICU staff do not typically follow patient outcomes after the ICU. Thankfully, this is changing as many hospitals develop special ICU aftercare clinics or recovery centers (e.g., www.icudelirium.org/the-icu-recovery-center-at-vanderbilt).

- Before discharge, get the contact information of an ICU doctor or nurse who can act as an information source for you and your post-ICU doctor(s).

- Request information on the side effects of any medication you are given during hospitalization and request prescriptions and refills before discharge. Discuss these medications with your health-care provider after discharge from the ICU.

- Ensure that you are given specific referrals for any post-ICU therapy you may need. This may include care by an array of talented people including an occupational and/or speech therapist, physiatrist, physical therapist, psychologist, psychiatrist, neurologist, pulmonologist, nutritionist, or social worker.

- A patient and family are commonly completely unaware that such support is needed or available. This is precisely the function of the interprofessional teams who staff ICU recovery centers.

Stay on Top of Your Financial Situation

- Make sure your health insurance is up-to-date. If it might expire in the foreseeable future, make backup plans (e.g., COBRA, Medicare, Medicaid, ACA).

- Consider using daily/weekly/monthly budgeting tools. Seek help from a financial adviser. Try to build in a cushion for unforeseen medical expenses.

- Many people find it necessary to reduce ongoing expenses where possible and even sell assets if they are fortunate enough to have them.

- Consider applying for disability and any other applicable insurance coverage (e.g., unemployment, workers' compensation). Ask your social worker (if you had one in the hospital who is willing to help or to connect you to someone following discharge) or your medical team to advocate for you by making phone calls or writing letters or emails on your behalf.

- Consider getting help with any financial tasks that you used to do but which may be overly challenging now (e.g., taxes).

Accept Yourself for Who You Are Now

- Acknowledge your "new normal" state and build yourself back up from there. This acknowledgment may involve a season of grieving. There will likely be times when you feel as if you are going backward in your recovery.

- Identify a PICS support group. Check with your hospital if they organize or know of one. See the list of websites I have provided near the end of this resources section and communicate with these motivated and passionate teams for guidance and Zoom membership options.

- Friends, family, and many doctors may not understand what you are experiencing, so consider seeing a therapist to help you adjust to your ICU hospitalization and illness and/or injury.

- Treat yourself well with plenty of sleep and, if you are able, challenging mental and physical exercises and a well-balanced diet as recommended by your health-care providers.

- Keep things in perspective: most people do not survive what you have overcome. Time can be a great healer, so every day you get through can be a step closer to getting better.

- Remember that you survived a challenging illness and that you can do hard things, but also show yourself compassion.

COGNITIVE AND MENTAL HEALTH REMEDIATION

Memory Impairments

- Talk to your doctor about medications that may be suitable for managing cognitive difficulties or fatigue, yet be aware there are no magic solutions.

- Organize detailed daily/weekly/monthly schedules and set alarm reminders for important tasks (e.g., on a smartphone). You may need someone to help you with this.

- Keep references and to-do lists handy (including lists of medications and emergency contacts).

- Consider treatment with an occupational therapist, a speech and language pathologist, or a rehabilitation psychologist. These professionals can help you learn cognitive strategies and develop a plan for maximizing your existing abilities.

- When you feel up to it, try different activities that challenge your memory and rebuild your brain's neurological circuits. For example, sign up for a free online class, try computerized cognitive rehabilitation approaches such as BrainHQ.com or akiliinter active.com, play math games such as sudoku, word games such as Scrabble, or learn a new language on one of the language apps.

Attention and Concentration Difficulties

- Consider getting a neuropsychological evaluation. It can help identify your specific cognitive and psychological strengths and limitations to guide your recovery. Such testing can also be helpful in explaining your condition to others, including family, friends, doctors, insurance providers, and future employers.

- Plan out the topics you want to cover ahead of time, whether it be for conversations or written communications.

- Try setting up a regular (preferably daily) schedule of focus-demanding mental games (e.g., chess, sudoku) and physical activities (such as juggling or yoga) after discussion with your medical team.

Organizational and Problem-Solving Challenges

- Make sure to have a failproof system in place for managing your medication and bill payments. Use a daily medication organizer, set up automatic refills and bill payments, and enlist the help of a trusted individual to assist with complex tasks as needed.

- Understand your weaknesses organizationally and work within them.

- If available, leverage information technology tools (smartphones, calculators, spreadsheets, spelling correctors, organization apps) and consider using noise-cancellation headsets.

- Factor in significantly more time than you used to when planning new tasks.

- Break projects down into their smallest components and then solve each one individually. Consider meeting with a cognitive remediation specialist or an occupational therapist.

Managing Your Moods

- Consider getting assessed for post-ICU PTSD, anxiety, or depression. Mood symptoms can exacerbate or be confused with memory lapses or other cognitive problems.

- Talk to your doctor about medications that can help you manage anxiety and depression. While psychiatrists often handle these medications, they are also overseen by internists, family practitioners, and nurse practitioners.

- As hard as it seems, try to engage in a regular (preferably daily) exercise regimen. This is very important! Start off with something that you can manage easily, even if it's just walking a few steps across your living room, and build up from there. Try yoga for beginners if you're up for it. Both aerobic exercise and strength training have been shown to help people improve cognition and to be physically healthier and less frail.

- If you can, try to go outside each day.

- Connect with friends and family as much as possible, however possible, even when it feels difficult. Try text and video messages, emails, phone calls, postcards.

- Meditation and mindfulness can be helpful for mood and cognition. There are many free apps you could try.

- Join a PICS support group.

Awareness Challenges

- If you are unsure if you are struggling with cognitive difficulties following an ICU stay, ask people close to you if they notice something different in your behavior or speech.

PHYSICAL REMEDIATION

ICU-Acquired Weakness

- Get referrals for physical and occupational therapy, as needed. Engage in these therapies as early and as often as possible.

- Prior to hospital discharge, you are likely to get a full physical-function assessment. Make sure that your physical and/or occupational therapist(s) gets a copy of that report.

- If you have ongoing shortness of breath, ask your doctor about getting pulmonary function tests (PFTs), which can detect persistent lung damage. In addition, the lungs may be spared, yet muscles and nerves may be damaged as part of your PICS. In that case, other testing could include electromyography and nerve-conduction studies as well as exercise-tolerance tests. Ask about lung and/or cardiac rehabilitation if possible.

Managing Fatigue

- Discuss with your doctor the potential benefits of various medications for managing fatigue. Some physicians may order blood tests to check for hormonal imbalances that can contribute to fatigue (e.g., thyroid, estrogen, testosterone, cortisol).

- Getting quality sleep is essential to managing fatigue. Develop healthy sleep habits and discuss possible medications that may assist in or disrupt your sleep.

- If you have nightmares, consider getting assessed for PTSD (see the "Cognitive and Mental Health Remediation" section).

- Get as much sleep as your body needs for recovery.

- Bear in mind that physical exercise, if you can manage it, is good for sleep.

Difficulties in Carrying Out Functions of Daily Life

- Ask your medical team about different physical exercises that require coordination and/or balance (e.g., yoga, dancing, interval training). These exercises may help some and may injure others, so be sure to seek personalized advice about these activities.

- Whatever activities you choose, start small and build gradually.

- If appropriate, discuss getting a vision and/or hearing test with your doctor.

- Remember to nourish your body with music, reading, exercise, healthy eating, social connections, time outdoors, and rest.

Debunking Myths about the Aging Brain*

Myth	Fact
You are born with all the neurons that your brain will ever have.	Neurons are continually created throughout your life in areas of the brain through neurogenesis.
You can't learn new things as you age.	Learning can happen at any age through cognitively stimulating activities such as meeting new people or trying new hobbies.
We don't know how the brain works.	In recent years researchers have made great strides in understanding the brain. Neuroscience is at the cusp of new and exciting breakthroughs.
Dementia is an inevitable consequence of old age.	Dementia is not a normal part of aging. There are big differences between typical age-related changes in the brain and those that are caused by disease.
Only young people can learn a new language.	While it is simpler for kids, being older does not stop you from learning a new language.
You are doomed to forget things as you age.	Remembering details is easier for some people than others, but this is true at all ages. Proven strategies can help you remember names, facts, etc. Simply paying closer attention can often help you remember better.
A person who has memory training never forgets.	Keep practicing your memory skills. "Use it or lose it" applies to memory training in the same way it applies to maintaining your physical health.

* Modified with permission from the AARP Global Council on Brain Health.

BOOSTING YOUR BRAIN HEALTH

After a hospitalization, be sure to take care of your brain as well as your body.*

- *Move:* Every day find ways to move safely. Even a little exercise is better than none. Walking, strength training, stretching, chair exercises, group activities, enjoying nature, using a gym when safe and permitted by your medical team, and even performing household chores are a few ways to increase activity levels.

- *Discover:* Make time in your day to laugh, learn, be curious, and be grateful.

- *Relax:* Find moments to disconnect from stress, forgive yourself and others, breathe deeply, and simplify your life when possible. Prioritize a consistent schedule of quality sleep each night.

- *Nourish:* Eat healthy foods and limit alcohol. Seek professional nutritional help and counseling when appropriate.

- *Connect:* Focus on building healthy friendships and supportive relationships during this vulnerable period of recovery rather than allowing yourself to be depleted by stressful interactions. Sometimes we forget that we have choices about how to spend our time. Try to stop and think about the space between what you are faced with each day and how you react to it. Your mind and body are in dire need of healing. You may find meaning in your community through activities such as volunteer work or faith-based groups.

---

* Modified with permission from the AARP Global Council on Brain Health.

HELPFUL WEBSITES

I have curated a list of websites that I hope you will find helpful in navigating the realities of the critical care experience. These websites provide information and guidance on a variety of topics including delirium, PTSD, depression, dementia, disability, PICS, sepsis, ARDS, the aging brain and brain health, sleep, recovery, ICU diaries, quality improvement, survivor support groups, wellness, and more.

- aacn.org
- aarp.org
- americandeliriumsociety.org
- ardsglobal.org
- covid19.criticalcarerecovery.com
- edinburghroyalinfirmary.criticalcarerecovery.com
- esicm.org
- europeandeliriumassociation.org
- geriacademy.com
- help.agscocare.org
- hopkinsmedicine.org/pulmonary/research/outcomes-after-critical-illness
- hospitalelderlifeprogram.org
- humanizingintensivecare.com
- ics.ac.uk
- icudelirium.org
- icu-diary.org/diary/Diary.html
- icusteps.org
- ihi.org
- nice.org.uk

Resources

- readingicusupport.co.uk/index.html
- sccm.org
- sepsis.org
- thoracic.org

Books to Explore

HERE IS A SHORT list of books (among dozens more) that inspired me during the genesis and writing of *Every Deep-Drawn Breath*.

- Abbey, Aoife, *Seven Signs of Life*
- Alexander, Michelle, *The New Jim Crow*
- Angelou, Maya, *I Know Why the Caged Bird Sings*
- Aronson, Louise, *Elderhood*
- Awdish, Rana, *In Shock*
- Blackmon, Douglas, *Slavery by Another Name*
- Bragg, Rick, *All Over but the Shoutin'*
- Brown, Brené, *The Gifts of Imperfection*
- Butler, Katy, *Knocking on Heaven's Door*
- Clarke, Rachel, *Dear Life*
- Collins, Jim, *Good to Great*
- Crimmins, Cathy, *Where Is the Mango Princess?*
- Day, Dorothy, *The Long Loneliness*
- Doidge, Norman, *The Brain That Changes Itself*
- Dostoyevsky, Fyodor, *The Idiot*
- Eagleman, David, *Livewired*
- Farmer, Paul, *To Repair the World*
- Fitzgerald, F. Scott, *The Great Gatsby*
- Gawande, Atul, *Being Mortal*

- Gladwell, Malcolm, *The Tipping Point*
- Hawking, Stephen, *A Brief History of Time*
- Hirshfield, Jane, *The October Palace*
- Kafka, Franz, *The Trial*
- Kahneman, Daniel, *Thinking, Fast and Slow*
- Kalanithi, Paul, *When Breath Becomes Air*
- Kandel, Eric, *The Age of Insight*
- Lamas, Daniela, *You Can Stop Humming Now*
- Lewis, C. S., *The Screwtape Letters*
- Lewis, Sinclair, *Arrowsmith*
- Maclean, Norman, *Young Men and Fire*
- McCullough, David, *John Adams*
- Miller, BJ, and Shoshana Berger, *A Beginner's Guide to the End*
- Mukherjee, Siddhartha, *The Emperor of All Maladies*
- Ofri, Danielle, *What Patients Say, What Doctors Hear*
- Osler, Sir William, "Aequanimitas"
- Patchett, Ann, *Bel Canto*
- Powell, Tia, *Dementia Reimagined*
- Puri, Sunita, *That Good Night*
- Sacks, Oliver, *Awakenings*
- Steinbeck, John, *East of Eden*
- Stevenson, Bryan, *Just Mercy*
- Verghese, Abraham, *My Own Country*
- Volandes, Angelo, *The Conversation*
- Zitter, Jessica, *Extreme Measures*

Acknowledgments

I'D LIKE TO THANK my family for their undying patience. Kim, my wife of well over thirty years and into eternity, always manages to find more love for me in her heart than I deserve. My three adult children have been subjected to more gory details of critical care than was probably smart of me to share. What's more, unless they were bleeding out, I never considered their physical injuries anything of concern. Somewhat redemptive is that I was always willing to suture their lacerations or care for their burns when the unexpected happened on a camping trip or at a sporting event.

So many people selflessly gave of themselves to help me write this book. I was toying with the idea for over ten years, and along the way a boatload of wisdom was poured down on me. One pearl was the importance of patience along the path of scientific discovery. We hoe a very long row in academics, and clarity only comes with the passage of years and the acquisition of gray hair. To wit, I'd like to thank my mentors Dr. Joan W. Bennett, Dr. Edward F. Haponik, Dr. William R. Hazzard, Dr. Gordon R. Bernard, and Dr. Robert S. Dittus. From them I learned more than methodology and data analysis. They taught me a proper priority list and how to walk forward, though I admit I tripped along the way.

I want to thank the people who shaped my life goal of becoming a physician. Amid the sweat and heat of my childhood working in the fields, slogging in the bayou for crawfish for dinner, learning in the classrooms, at the youth shelter my mom directed, the individuals who took the time to let me watch and listen to them. It would be impossible to name them all, but I remember them each in a special way.

Thanks to the men who stepped into my life when my single mom was doing her best to raise my brother, Scott, sister, Erin, and me. I found a stalwart father figure in my uncle Warren C. Lowe, who introduced me to the bright worlds of artists such as Clementine Hunter and James Harold Jennings. Thanks to my father-in-law, Frank Adams, whom I called Dad. To Gene Ely, my deceased father, thank you for your love of me. I looked up to you more than you ever knew.

Thanks to family treasures Greg and Nanny for keeping me laughing at *I Love Lucy* reruns. To Dr. Sarah Corser, my sister by Gwen Ely, your family is a reflection of light. You and my brother-in-law, Noel, are living out my other dream of being a country doctor.

Similarly, I'd like to thank the countless nurses, physicians, PharmDs, physician assistants, nurse practitioners, physical and occupational therapists, respiratory therapists, nutritionists, social workers, and hospital chaplains who day by day imparted their knowledge into my life and practice. With each of them, we shared a patient who taught me as well. Thank you all. This book is your story.

Our research is built on the firm footing of the Veterans Administration, the National Institutes of Health, the American Federation for Aging Research, and other foundations who review our grants and award us funding to make our dream of addressing hypotheses a reality. I want to extend particular thanks to R. Luci Roberts, PhD, Susan J. Zieman, MD, PhD, and Molly V. Wagster, PhD, who work tirelessly alongside a huge team of others at the National Institute on Aging for all of us in the field of delirium and dementia research at a national and international level to advance the science and improve the lives of countless patients. I find few things as exciting as asking a question no one knows the answer to and then following a methodical path to the answer. My colleagues and I at the CIBS Center always say we don't care what we learn, as long as it is the truth. Each person at our center works tirelessly to enroll patients, collect and analyze data carefully, and then get the word out to help patients we'll never meet. For each of you, patients included of course, I am thankful. It's a big, messy family.

Academia is a family as well. How many times have I been challenged at a podium or in a scientific congress and forced to muster defense for a proposed change to standard care? How many times have these calibrations led me to reconsider, take a few steps back, and start again from a better vantage point? This academic process is extremely humbling, and through it we all develop very thick skin. Yet the many facets of peer review are time-tested, and they work. We care enough about patients and science itself to push each other to do better. Ultimately, this is how all of medicine continues to be transformed. To each person who demanded more of me, I thank you for influencing me along the way.

To Lindsey Tate, my incessant collaborator and partner in writing this book, words can't adequately convey my appreciation. From our love of Dostoyevsky, we went forward. I still laugh at our joke about feeling at times as if we were trying to stuff a huge sleeping bag of information into a pouch that was too small. You always sought the theme of maintaining our gaze on the person in the patient, and it served as our North Star.

Susan Golomb, my agent, your dogged enthusiasm, insights, and powerful persona drove me. Thank you not only for your encyclopedic knowledge of the book world, but also for your kind admonishments to me to be careful on the front lines during the pandemic. I know it came from a sincere place of caring for me as a person. Kara Watson, my editor at Scribner, and Nan Graham, my publisher, who saw the vision of this book during the COVID-19 pandemic: thank you for taking a chance on a new author and for believing in the larger purpose of my work. Kara, I'm grateful for your unflagging patience, insights, and uncanny instincts that edified me along the way.

I would also like to thank three readers of the original manuscript who offered thoughtful comments: Dr. Hannah Wunsch and Dr. Angelo Volandes shared their medical expertise, while Sister Nena DeMatteo— who taught my daughters (and Ann Patchett) how to read—lent her finely tuned ear for language.

At each phase of my life, I have had gifted spiritual advisers. E. J. Jacques, SJ, had me dive into the golden braid of *Gödel, Escher, Bach* in high school and kept me rooted. Brother Dubba Marion, my uncle Dubba, gave me reprieve at St. Joseph Abbey in Saint Benedict, Louisiana, during long weekends in medical school. Richard C. Hermes, SJ, I am still rejuvenated by our covert high school exchanges of lyrics from Bob Dylan's *Blood on the Tracks*. John J. Raphael, BCC, my best friend in Nashville, thank you for always being there to guide me when I didn't know where to go next. And Bill W., I am among the legions of people you have saved. My Al-Anon sponsor, whom I also thank, would attest to that.

I want to thank dear friends for helping me even when you didn't know it. An incomplete list includes Mary, Teresa, Catherine, Faustina, Therese, Bakhita, Gianna, Joseph, Francis, Thomas, Ignatius, and John. Let me not forget GK, Jacques, Flannery, Caryll, Alexander, Franz, Fulton, and Walter.

Finally, the main reason I wrote this book was to do everything possible to ensure that future patients get the best care, have the most complete recovery, and have the most peaceful death when their lives reach a natural end. Therefore, I am donating my book advance as well any additional royalties I may receive from this book (net of agency fees) to a fund at the CIBS Center devoted to cutting-edge research about critical illness, promoting the widespread adoption of evidence-based practices, and helping ICU survivors and their families. I am the codirector of the CIBS Center, and I encourage you to learn more and to consider a donation by visiting our website, www.icudelirium.org.

Notes

Epigraph

vii   East of Eden: J. Steinbeck, *East of Eden* (Penguin, 2002).

Prologue

2   *Charity Hospital, a 250-year-old refuge:* J. E. Salvaggio, *New Orleans' Charity Hospital: A Story of Physicians, Politics, and Poverty* (LSU Press, 1992).

4   *"We got a future . . .":* J. Steinbeck. *Of Mice and Men* (Penguin, 1993), 14.

11   *more than 6 million patients will land in intensive care each year:* E. Milbrandt, R. Watson, F. Mayr, et al., "How Big Is Critical Care in the US?," *Critical Care Medicine* 36 (2008): A77; and C. M. Coopersmith, H. Wunsch, M. P. Fink, et al., "A Comparison of Critical Care Research Funding and the Financial Burden of Critical Illness in the United States," *Critical Care Medicine* 40 (2012): 1072–79.

Chapter 1: Fractured Lives—Embracing a New Normal

15   *post-intensive care syndrome (PICS):* D. M. Needham, J. Davidson, H. Cohen, et al., "Improving Long-Term Outcomes

after Discharge from Intensive Care Unit: Report from a Stakeholders' Conference," *Critical Care Medicine* 40 (2012): 502–9; and J. L. Stollings, S. L. Bloom, E. L. Huggins, et al., "Medication Management to Ameliorate Post-Intensive Care Syndrome," *AACN Advanced Critical Care* 27 (2016): 133–40.

16   *Critical Illness, Brain Dysfunction, and Survivorship (CIBS) Center:* Critical Illness, Brain Dysfunction, and Survivorship (CIBS) Center for ICU Delirium and Dementia, 2020, https://www .icudelirium.org/.

20   *Wechsler Adult Intelligence Scale:* D. Wechsler, *Wechsler Adult Intelligence Scale Manual,* 3rd ed. (*WAIS-III*) (Psychological Corporation, 1997).

24   *one in five ICU survivors develops PTSD, and one in three develops depression and anxiety:* J. C. Jackson, P. P. Pandharipande, T. D. Girard, et al., "Depression, Post-Traumatic Stress Disorder, and Functional Disability in Survivors of Critical Illness in the BRAIN-ICU Study: A Longitudinal Cohort Study," *Lancet Respiratory Medicine* 2, no. 3 (2014): 369–79.

25   *suffering with PICS haven't returned to work:* B. C. Norman, J. C. Jackson, J. A. Graves, et al., "Employment Outcomes after Critical Illness: An Analysis of the Bringing to Light the Risk Factors and Incidence of Neuropsychological Dysfunction in ICU Survivors Cohort," *Critical Care Medicine* 44 (2016): 2003–9.

25   *It's a family disease, and we refer to it as PICS-F:* J. E. Davidson, C. Jones, and O. J. Bienvenu, "Family Response to Critical Illness: Postintensive Care Syndrome—Family," *Critical Care Medicine* 40 (2012): 618–24.

Chapter 2: Early History of Critical Care—Bumpy Gravel Roads to ICU Interstates

27   *"I was taught that the way":* M. Curie, V. L. Kellogg, and C. Kellogg, *Pierre Curie* (Macmillan, 1923), 167.

30   *It costs about $2,000 to $4,000 per square foot to build a modern ICU room:* D. Angus, personal communication, March 20, 2020.

31   *In the United States alone, we spend more than $3 trillion:* "How We Spend $3,400,000,000,000," *The Atlantic*, 2017, https:// www.theatlantic.com/health/archive/2017/06/how-we-spend -3400000000000/530355/.

31   *that figure is projected to rise to approximately one-fifth of our entire GDP:* "Healthcare Spending Will Hit 19.4% of GDP in the Next Decade, CMS Projects," Modern Health Care, 2019, https://www .modernhealthcare.com/article/20190220/NEWS/190229989 /healthcare-spending-will-hit-19-4-of-gdp-in-the-next-decade-cms -projects; and "Healthcare Spending Near 20 Percent of GDP, More Than Any Other Country," Health Care Finance News, 2018, https://www.healthcarefinancenews.com/news/healthcare -spending-near-20-percent-gdp-more-any-other-country.

31   *the proportion of these that are ICU beds has steadily escalated:* N. A. Halpern, D. A. Goldman, K. S. Tan, et al., "Trends in Critical Care Beds and Use among Population Groups and Medicare and Medicaid Beneficiaries in the United States: 2000–2010," *Critical Care Medicine* 44 (2016): 1490–99.

32   *25 million days in ICUs in the United States:* N. A. Halpern and S. M. Pastores, "Critical Care Medicine in the United States, 2000–2005: An Analysis of Bed Numbers, Occupancy Rates, Payer Mix, and Costs," *Critical Care Medicine* 38 (2010): 65–71; and SCCM Critical Care Statistics, 2020, https://sccm.org /Communications/Critical-Care-Statistics.

32   *one-third reduction in the likelihood of death for ICU patients:*
J. E. Zimmerman, A. A. Kramer, and W. A. Knaus, "Changes in
Hospital Mortality for United States Intensive Care Unit Admissions
from 1988 to 2012," *Critical Care* 17 (2013): R81.

33   *But not until the 1970s did such rooms become commonplace in US
hospitals:* M. Hilberman, "The Evolution of Intensive Care Units,"
Critical Care Medicine 3 (1975): 159–65.

35   *Copenhagen's polio epidemic ballooned to nine hundred patients:*
H. C. Lassen, "A Preliminary Report on the 1952 Epidemic of
Poliomyelitis in Copenhagen with Special Reference to the Treat-
ment of Acute Respiratory Insufficiency," *Lancet* 1 (1953): 37–41.

39   *soon intensive care units were springing up in hospitals across
the country:* P. Safar and A. Grenvik, "Critical Care Medicine.
Organizing and Staffing Intensive Care Units," *Chest* 59
(1971): 535–47; and M. Weil and H. Shubin, "The
New Practice of Critical Care Medicine," *Chest* 59 (1971):
473–74.

Chapter 3: Culture of Critical Care—The Era of Deep Sedation and Immobilization

49   *Guyton's classic physiology textbook:* A. C. Guyton and J. E. Hall,
Human Physiology and Mechanisms of Disease (Saunders, 1987);
and A. Guyton and J. Hall, *Guyton and Hall: Textbook of Medical
Physiology,* 13th ed. (Saunders, 2017).

51   *the first lung transplant in a human:* J. D. Hardy, W. R. Webb,
M. L. Dalton Jr., et al., "Lung Homotransplantation in Man,"
JAMA 186 (1963): 1065–74.

52   *this lifesaving intervention was discovered through sheer luck:*
B. E. Levine, "Fifty Years of Research in ARDS. ARDS: How It All

Began," *American Journal of Respiratory and Critical Care Medicine* 196 (2017): 1247–48.

52   *condition would be defined by Petty, the following year, as adult respiratory distress syndrome:* D. G. Ashbaugh, D. B. Bigelow, T. L. Petty, et al., "Acute Respiratory Distress in Adults," *Lancet* 2 (1967): 319–23.

Chapter 4: The World of Transplant Medicine— Harvesting the Right Path Forward

57   *"paralyzed, sedated patients, lying without motion, appearing to be dead":* T. L. Petty, "Suspended Life or Extending Death?," *Chest* 114 (1998): 360–61.

59   *John Russell, was a hospitalized prison inmate:* W. Vigneswaran, E. Garrity, and J. Odell, *Lung Transplantation: Principles and Practice* (CRC Press, 2016).

59   *took his last breath in the same hospital's emergency room:* M. L. Dalton, "The First Lung Transplantation," *Annals of Thoracic Surgery* 60 (1995): 1437–38.

66   *chief-resident research project in the* New England Journal of Medicine: E. W. Ely, A. M. Baker, D. P. Dunagan, et al., "Effect on the Duration of Mechanical Ventilation of Identifying Patients Capable of Breathing Spontaneously," *New England Journal of Medicine* 335 (1996): 1864–69.

66   *study focused on the creation of a weaning standard:* I had been inspired by the recent work of Dr. Laurent Brochard, a Parisian intensivist, who had proved that a new type of tight-fitting mask that pushed air into the lungs—a bilevel positive airway pressure (BiPAP) mask—could obviate time on a ventilator for patients and save their lives. My SBT study complemented and

built on the pioneering work of Dr. Martin Tobin from Chicago and a famous Spanish lung doctor, Andrés Esteban. Their three papers are as follows: L. Brochard, J. Mancebo, M. Wysocki, et al., "Noninvasive Ventilation for Acute Exacerbations of Chronic Obstructive Pulmonary Disease," *New England Journal of Medicine* 333 (1995): 817–22; K. L. Yang and M. J. Tobin, "A Prospective Study of Indexes Predicting the Outcome of Trials of Weaning from Mechanical Ventilation," *New England Journal of Medicine* 324 (1991): 1445–50; and A. Esteban, F. Frutos, M. J. Tobin, et al., "A Comparison of Four Methods of Weaning Patients from Mechanical Ventilation. Spanish Lung Failure Collaborative Group," *New England Journal of Medicine* 332 (1995): 345–50.

67   *blue skin, then purple lips:* E. W. Ely, "A Piece of My Mind. Cyanosis," *JAMA* 305 (2011): 2388–89.

72   *sporting a leopard-skin bra:* E. W. Ely, "A Piece of My Mind. The Leopard-Skin Bra," *JAMA* 305 (2011): 756–57.

Chapter 5: Delirium Disaster—An Invisible Calamity for Patients and Families

78   *first used for delirium in critically ill patients in 1973 when Dr. Edwin "Ned" Cassem:* N. Cassem, "Intravenous Use of Haloperidol for Acute Delirium in Intensive Care Settings," *Continuing Medical Education Syllabus and Scientific Proceedings in Summary Form,* no. 394 (from the 131st Annual Meeting of the American Psychiatric Association, Washington, DC, 1978), 204–5.

79   *I had dismissed this as ICU psychosis:* G. Fricchione, "What Is an ICU Psychosis?," *Harvard Mental Health Letter* 16 (1999): 7.

79   *Drs. George Engel and John Romano from the* Journal of Neuropsychiatry *in 1959:* G. L. Engel and J. Romano, "Delirium, a

Syndrome of Cerebral Insufficiency," *Journal of Chronic Diseases* 9 (1959): 260–77.

81   *something other than their lungs was causing older ones to die:* E. W. Ely, G. W. Evans, and E. F. Haponik, "Mechanical Ventilation in a Cohort of Elderly Patients Admitted to an Intensive Care Unit," *Annals of Internal Medicine* 131 (1999): 96–104.

83   *Eric Kandel and James Schwartz's* Principles of Neural Science*:* E. R. Kandel, J. H. Schwartz, T. M. Jessell, et al., *Principles of Neural Science*, 2nd ed. (Amsterdam, Netherlands: Elsevier Science, 1985).

84   *building on work by Dr. Sharon Inouye:* S. K. Inouye, C. H. van Dyck, C. A. Alessi, et al., "Clarifying Confusion: The Confusion Assessment Method. A New Method for Detection of Delirium," *Annals of Internal Medicine* 113 (1990): 941–48.

84   *In our first delirium study, Brenda and I enrolled 111 patients:* E. W. Ely, S. K. Inouye, G. R. Bernard, et al., "Delirium in Mechanically Ventilated Patients: Validity and Reliability of the Confusion Assessment Method for the Intensive Care Unit (CAM-ICU)," *JAMA* 286 (2001): 2703–10; and E. W. Ely, R. Margolin, J. Francis, et al., "Evaluation of Delirium in Critically Ill Patients: Validation of the Confusion Assessment Method for the Intensive Care Unit (CAM-ICU)," *Critical Care Medicine* 29 (2001): 1370–79.

86   *"Never be so focused":* Ann Patchett, *State of Wonder* (Harper Perennial, 2012), 246.

86   *CAM-ICU method was published in the* Journal of the American Medical Association*:* Ely et al., "Delirium in Mechanically Ventilated Patients."

86   *translated into over thirty-five languages:* "CAM-ICU Translations," 2020, https://www.icudelirium.org/medical-professionals/downloads/resource-language-translations.

86   *the Intensive Care Delirium Screening Checklist:* N. Bergeron, M. J. Dubois, M. Dumont, et al., "Intensive Care Delirium Screening Checklist: Evaluation of a New Screening Tool," *Intensive Care Medicine* 27 (2001): 859–64.

90   *We know so much more about delirium now:* J. E. Wilson, M. F. Mart, C. Cunningham, et al., "Delirium," *Nature Reviews Disease Primers* 6 (2020): 90.

93   *reduced delirium in older hospitalized (non-ICU) patients:* S. K. In- ouye, S. T. Bogardus Jr., P. A. Charpentier, et al., "A Multicomponent Intervention to Prevent Delirium in Hospitalized Older Patients," *New England Journal of Medicine* 340 (1999): 669–76.

94   *During the coronavirus pandemic, a lack of family:* R. Awd- ish and E. W. Ely, "Keeping Loved Ones from Visiting Our Coronavirus Patients Is Making Them Sicker," *Washington Post,* August 6, 2020; and B. T. Pun, R. Badenes, G. Heras La Calle, et al., "Prevalence and Risk Factors for Delirium in Critically Ill Patients with COVID-19 (COVID-D): A Multicentre Cohort Study," *Lancet* 9 (2021): 239–50.

Chapter 7: Deciding My Path—Combining Research with Clinical Care

104   *Delirium in the ICU predicted a higher likelihood of dying:* E. W. Ely, A. Shintani, B. Truman, et al., "Delirium as a Predictor of Mortal- ity in Mechanically Ventilated Patients in the Intensive Care Unit," *JAMA* 291 (2004): 1753–62.

105   *with stories of the infamous Angola:* A. Woodfox, *Solitary* (Grove Press, 2019).

107   *Richard Feynman, the brilliant physicist:* R. P. Feynman, "The Value of Science," *Engineering and Science* 19 (1955): 13–15; and Rich-

ard P. Feynman, *The Pleasure of Finding Things Out: The Best Short Works of Richard P. Feynman* (Basic Books, 1999).

Chapter 8: Unshackling the Brain—Finding Consciousness in the ICU

116   *paper on ethics consultations in the ICU:* L. J. Schneiderman, T. Gilmer, H. D. Teetzel, et al., "Effect of Ethics Consultations on Nonbeneficial Life-Sustaining Treatments in the Intensive Care Setting: A Randomized Controlled Trial," *JAMA* 290 (2003): 1166–72.

118   *ABC (Awakening and Breathing Controlled) trial:* T. D. Girard, J. P. Kress, B. D. Fuchs, et al., "Efficacy and Safety of a Paired Sedation and Ventilator Weaning Protocol for Mechanically Ventilated Patients in Intensive Care (Awakening and Breathing Controlled Trial): A Randomised Controlled Trial," *Lancet* 371 (2008): 126–34.

118   *MENDS (Maximizing Efficacy of Targeted Sedation and Reducing Neurological Dysfunction) trial:* P. P. Pandharipande, B. T. Pun, D. L. Herr, et al., "Effect of Sedation with Dexmedetomidine vs. Lorazepam on Acute Brain Dysfunction in Mechanically Ventilated Patients: The MENDS Randomized Controlled Trial," *JAMA* 298 (2007): 2644–53.

118   *my first study, in which we turned off the ventilator:* E. W. Ely, A. M. Baker, D. P. Dunagan, et al., "Effect on the Duration of Mechanical Ventilation of Identifying Patients Capable of Breathing Spontaneously," *New England Journal of Medicine* 335 (1996): 1864–69.

118   *Drs. J. P. Kress and Jesse Hall, who had pioneered shutting off sedation:* J. P. Kress, A. S. Pohlman, M. F. O'Connor, et al., "Daily Interruption of Sedative Infusions in Critically Ill Patients

Undergoing Mechanical Ventilation," *New England Journal of Medicine* 342 (2000): 1471–77.

118   *most prescribed drugs in the world:* A. M. Washton and J. E. Zweben, *Treating Alcohol and Drug Problems in Psychotherapy Practice: Doing What Works* (Guilford Press, 2006), 47.

119   *"I was now the dying man":* S. Bellow, *Ravelstein* (Penguin, 2006), 180.

121   *Dr. Edmond "Ted" Eger developed a clinical tool:* G. Merkel and E. I. Eger, 2nd, "A Comparative Study of Halothane and Halopropane Anesthesia Including Method for Determining Equipotency," *Anesthesiology* 24 (1963): 346–57; and E. I. Eger, 2nd, "A Brief History of the Origin of Minimum Alveolar Concentration (MAC)," *Anesthesiology* 96 (2002): 238–39.

121   *the Ramsay scale:* M. A. Ramsay, T. M. Savege, B. R. Simpson, et al., "Controlled Sedation with Alphaxalone-Alphadolone," *British Medical Journal* 2 (1974): 656–59.

121   *Richmond Agitation-Sedation Scale (RASS):* C. N. Sessler, M. S. Gosnell, M. J. Grap, et al., "The Richmond Agitation-Sedation Scale: Validity and Reliability in Adult Intensive Care Unit Patients," *American Journal of Respiratory and Critical Care Medicine* 166 (2002): 1338–44.

121   *Sedation Agitation Scale (SAS):* R. R. Riker, J. T. Picard, and G. L. Fraser, "Prospective Evaluation of the Sedation-Agitation Scale for Adult Critically Ill Patients," *Critical Care Medicine* 27 (1999): 1325–29.

121   *we designed and completed a large study to revalidate and integrate the RASS:* E. W. Ely, B. Truman, A. Shintani, et al., "Monitoring Sedation Status over Time in ICU Patients: Reliability and Validity of the Richmond Agitation-Sedation Scale (RASS)," *JAMA* 289 (2003): 2983–91.

126 *burst suppression was a predictor of higher death rates:* P. L. Watson, A. K. Shintani, R. Tyson, et al., "Presence of Electroencephalogram Burst Suppression in Sedated, Critically Ill Patients Is Associated with Increased Mortality," *Critical Care Medicine* 36 (2008): 3171–77.

126 *Cook had studied 851 patients in Canada:* D. Cook, G. Rocker, J. Marshall, et al., "Withdrawal of Mechanical Ventilation in Anticipation of Death in the Intensive Care Unit," *New England Journal of Medicine* 349 (2003): 1123–32.

129 *forty-four ICUs across France:* J. F. Payen, G. Chanques, J. Mantz, et al., "Current Practices in Sedation and Analgesia for Mechanically Ventilated Critically Ill Patients: A Prospective Multicenter Patient-Based Study," *Anesthesiology* 106 (2007): 687–95.

129 *standard practice of using benzos:* Pandharipande et al., "Effect of Sedation with Dexmedetomidine."

129 *we learned that being awake on a ventilator did not increase psychological injury:* J. C. Jackson, T. D. Girard, S. M. Gordon, et al., "Long-Term Cognitive and Psychological Outcomes in the Awakening and Breathing Controlled Trial," *American Journal of Respiratory and Critical Care Medicine* 182 (2010): 183–91.

131 *This practice actually increased the likelihood of her dying:* Acute Respiratory Distress Syndrome Network, "Ventilation with Lower Tidal Volumes as Compared with Traditional Tidal Volumes for Acute Lung Injury and the Acute Respiratory Distress Syndrome," *New England Journal of Medicine* 342 (2000): 1301–8.

Chapter 9: Awakening Change—Patients Are Resurfacing

133   *"no sedation" protocol in their ICU patients on ventilators:*
T. Strøm, T. Martinussen, and P. Toft, "A Protocol of No Seda-
tion for Critically Ill Patients Receiving Mechanical Ventilation:
A Randomised Trial," *Lancet* 375 (2010): 475–80.

135   *Patients seemed better able to handle their fears:* J. P. Kress,
B. Gehlbach, M. Lacy, et al., "The Long-Term Psychological
Effects of Daily Sedative Interruption on Critically Ill Patients,"
American Journal of Respiratory and Critical Care Medicine 168
(2003): 1457–61; and J. C. Jackson, T. D. Girard, S. M. Gordon, et al., "Long-Term Cognitive and Psychological Outcomes
in the Awakening and Breathing Controlled Trial," *American
Journal of Respiratory and Critical Care Medicine* 182 (2010):
183–91.

137   *"Sometimes a kind of glory":* J. Steinbeck, *East of Eden* (Penguin,
2002), 131.

138   *They had coined the term* post-intensive care syndrome *(PICS):*
D. M. Needham, J. Davidson, H. Cohen, et al., "Improving
Long-Term Outcomes after Discharge from Intensive Care Unit:
Report from a Stakeholders' Conference," *Critical Care Medicine*
40 (2012): 502–9.

139   *five years after critical illness, survivors had difficulty:* M. S. Her-
ridge, C. M. Tansey, A. Matte, et al., "Functional Disability 5
Years after Acute Respiratory Distress Syndrome," *New England
Journal of Medicine* 364 (2011): 1293–304.

139   *landmark study on walking ventilated patients:* W. D. Schweickert, M. C. Pohlman, A. S. Pohlman, et al., "Early Physical and
Occupational Therapy in Mechanically Ventilated, Critically Ill

Patients: A Randomised Controlled Trial," *Lancet* 373 (2009): 1874–82.

140 *Just as Dr. Cook's* New England Journal of Medicine *paper had shown:* Cook et al., "Withdrawal of Mechanical Ventilation in Anticipation of Death in the Intensive Care Unit."

142 *"Scientists, too, as J. Robert Oppenheimer once remarked":* R. Solnit, *A Field Guide to Getting Lost* (Penguin, 2006).

143 *Dr. Jodi Halpern's work on clinical empathy:* J. Halpern, *From Detached Concern to Empathy: Humanizing Medical Practice* (Oxford University Press, 2001).

150 *"When I recovered from my pneumonia":* Steinbeck, *East of Eden*, 150.

151 *British doctor, Richard Griffiths, at various conferences, and one of his classic papers:* R. D. Griffiths and J. B. Hall, "Intensive Care Unit–Acquired Weakness," *Critical Care Medicine* 38 (2010): 779–87; and R. D. Griffiths and C. Jones, "Seven Lessons from 20 Years of Follow-Up of Intensive Care Unit Survivors," *Current Opinion in Critical Care* 13 (2007): 508–13.

152 *where he biopsied muscles:* R. Edwards, A. Young, and M. Wiles, "Needle Biopsy of Skeletal Muscle in the Diagnosis of Myopathy and the Clinical Study of Muscle Function and Repair," *New England Journal of Medicine* 302 (1980): 261–71.

153 *the immobilized leg had profound muscle degeneration:* R. D. Griffiths, T. E. Palmer, T. Helliwell, et al., "Effect of Passive Stretching on the Wasting of Muscle in the Critically Ill," *Nutrition* 11 (1995): 428–32.

Chapter 10: Spreading the Word—Putting New Ideas into Practice

157 *BRAIN-ICU investigation had proved it:* P. P. Pandharipande, T. D. Girard, J. C. Jackson, et al., "Long-Term Cognitive Impairment after Critical Illness," *New England Journal of Medicine* 369 (2013): 1306–16.

158 *never been able to shake the image of Sarah Beth's post-ICU brain:* J. C. Jackson, S. M. Gordon, D. Burger, et al., "Acute Respiratory Distress Syndrome and Long-Term Cognitive Impairment: A Case Study," *Archives of Clinical Neuropsychology* 18 (2003): 688.

158 *neuroimaging program, called VISIONS:* A. Morandi, B. P. Rogers, M. L. Gunther, et al., "The Relationship between Delirium Duration, White Matter Integrity, and Cognitive Impairment in Intensive Care Unit Survivors as Determined by Diffusion Tensor Imaging: The VISIONS Prospective Cohort Magnetic Resonance Imaging Study," *Critical Care Medicine* 40 (2012): 2182–89; and M. L. Gunther, A. Morandi, E. Krauskopf, et al., "The Association between Brain Volumes, Delirium Duration, and Cognitive Outcomes in Intensive Care Unit Survivors: The VISIONS Cohort Magnetic Resonance Imaging Study," *Critical Care Medicine* 40 (2012): 2022–32.

161 *(CTE), a dementia that develops in many retired professional football players:* B. I. Omalu, R. L. Hamilton, M. I. Kamboh, et al., "Chronic Traumatic Encephalopathy (CTE) in a National Football League Player: Case Report and Emerging Medicolegal Practice Questions," *Journal of Forensic Nursing* 6 (2010): 40–46; B. Omalu, J. Bailes, R. L. Hamilton, et al., "Emerging Histomorphologic Phenotypes of Chronic Traumatic Encephalopathy in American Athletes," *Neurosurgery* 69 (2011): 173–83, discussion, 83; and J. Mez, D. H. Daneshvar, P. T. Kiernan, et al., "Clinicopathological Evaluation of Chronic Traumatic Encephalopathy in Players of American Football," *JAMA* 318 (2017): 360–70.

162   *I knew this from extensive studies:* D. J. Emanuel, D. L. Fair-
clough, and L. L. Emanuel, "Attitudes and Desires Related to
Euthanasia and Physician-Assisted Suicide among Terminally
Ill Patients and Their Caregivers," *JAMA* 284 (2000): 2460–68;
and E. W. Ely, "What Happens When a Patient Says, 'Doc,
Help Me Die,'" CNN, March 20, 2018, https://www.cnn
.com/2018/03/20/opinions/caregiving-what-its-like-to-be-me
-wes-ely-opinion/index.html.

162   *benzos were strong predictors of the development of delirium:*
P. Pandharipande, A. Shintani, J. Peterson, et al., "Lorazepam
Is an Independent Risk Factor for Transitioning to Delirium in
Intensive Care Unit Patients," *Anesthesiology* 104 (2006): 21–26;
Pandharipande et al., "Long-Term Cognitive Impairment"; and
T. D. Girard, J. C. Jackson, P. P. Pandharipande, et al., "Delirium
as a Predictor of Long-Term Cognitive Impairment in Survivors
of Critical Illness," *Critical Care Medicine* 38 (2010): 1513–20.

162   *in twenty-seven studies over twenty-five years:* E. W. Ely, R. S.
Dittus, and T. D. Girard, "Point: Should Benzodiazepines Be
Avoided in Mechanically Ventilated Patients? Yes," *Chest* 142
(2012): 281–84; and E. W. Ely, R. S. Dittus, and T. D. Girard,
"Rebuttal from Dr. Ely et al.," *Chest* 142 (2012): 287–89.

163   *only 0.2 percent of ventilated patients were being walked:* P. Nydahl,
A. P. Ruhl, G. Bartoszek, et al., "Early Mobilization of Mechani-
cally Ventilated Patients: A 1-Day Point-Prevalence Study in
Germany," *Critical Care Medicine* 42 (2014): 1178–86.

164   *"It is to be measured by the quality of lives preserved or restored":*
G. Dunstan, "Hard Questions in Intensive Care: A Moralist An-
swers Questions Put to Him at a Meeting of the Intensive Care
Society, Autumn, 1984," *Anaesthesia* 40 (1985): 479–82.

166   *Dr. Donald Berwick . . . delivered a memorable speech:* D. M.
Berwick, *Escape Fire: Designs for the Future of Health Care* (John

Wiley & Sons, 2010); and "Escape Fire: Don Berwick National
Forum Address, 1999."

166   *"Rethinking Critical Care":* R. Bassett, K. M. Adams, V. Danesh,
       et al., "Rethinking Critical Care: Decreasing Sedation, Increasing
       Delirium Monitoring, and Increasing Patient Mobility," *Joint Com-
       mission Journal on Quality and Patient Safety* 41 (2015): 62–74.

167   *this means bridging the chasm between the care we* are *getting:*
       "Crossing the Quality Chasm," IHI, 2020, http://www.ihi.org
       /resources/Pages/Publications/CrossingtheQualityChasmA
       NewHealthSystemforthe21stCentury.aspx.

167   *Dr. Avedis Donabedian, the father of quality assessment:* A. Don-
       abedian, "The Quality of Care. How Can It Be Assessed?," *JAMA*
       260 (1988): 1743–48.

168   *upon the foundation of our own ABC* Lancet *study:* Girard et al.,
       "Efficacy and Safety of a Paired Sedation and Ventilator Wean-
       ing Protocol for Mechanically Ventilated Patients in Intensive
       Care (Awakening and Breathing Controlled Trial)."

168   *In the spirit of Malcolm Gladwell's* The Tipping Point*:* M. Glad-
       well, *The Tipping Point* (Little, Brown, 2000).

171   *Sutter Health hospital teams enrolled 6,064 patients:* M. A.
       Barnes-Daly, G. Phillips, and E. W. Ely, "Improving Hospital
       Survival and Reducing Brain Dysfunction at Seven California
       Community Hospitals: Implementing PAD Guidelines via the
       ABCDEF Bundle in 6,064 Patients," *Critical Care Medicine* 45
       (2017): 171–78.

173   *ICU Liberation Collaborative of the Society of Critical Care Medi-
       cine:* E. W. Ely, "The ABCDEF Bundle: Science and Philosophy
       of How ICU Liberation Serves Patients and Families," *Critical
       Care Medicine* 45 (2017): 321–30; and "ICU Liberation Initia-

tive," Society of Critical Care Medicine, 2020, https://sccm.org/ICULiberation/About.

175   *the more the entire A2F bundle was employed, the less time patients:* B. T. Pun, M. C. Balas, M. A. Barnes-Daly, et al., "Caring for Critically Ill Patients with the ABCDEF Bundle: Results of the ICU Liberation Collaborative in Over 15,000 Adults," *Critical Care Medicine* 47 (2019): 3–14.

175   *National Institute on Aging–sponsored MIND-USA study:* T. D. Girard, M. C. Exline, S. S. Carson, et al., "Haloperidol and Ziprasidone for Treatment of Delirium in Critical Illness," *New England Journal of Medicine* 379 (2018): 2506–16.

175   *six steps of the A2F bundle:* Critical Illness, Brain Dysfunction, and Survivorship (CIBS) Center for ICU Delirium and Dementia, 2020, https://www.icudelirium.org/.

176   *When we conducted a survey:* A. Morandi, S. Piva, E. W. Ely, et al., "Worldwide Survey of the 'Assessing Pain, Both Spontaneous Awakening and Breathing Trials, Choice of Drugs, Delirium Monitoring/Management, Early Exercise/Mobility, and Family Empowerment' (ABCDEF) Bundle," *Critical Care Medicine* 45 (2017): e1111–22.

178   *We used light sedation:* Y. Shehabi, R. Bellomo, M. Reade, et al., "Early Intensive Care Sedation Predicts Long-Term Mortality in Ventilated Critically Ill Patients," *American Journal of Respiratory and Critical Care Medicine* 186 (2012): 724–31; and C. G. Hughes, P. T. Mailloux, J. W. Devlin, et al., "MENDS2 Study Investigators. Dexmedetomidine or Propofol for Sedation in Mechanically Ventilated Adults with Sepsis," *New England Journal of Medicine* 384 (2021): 1424–36.

178   *I reread Avedis Donabedian's work on quality improvement:* F. Mullan, "A Founder of Quality Assessment Encounters a Troubled System Firsthand," *Health Affairs* 20, no. 1 (2001): 137–41.

Chapter 11: Finding the Person in the Patient—
Hope through Humanization

180   *Humanizing Intensive Care project (Proyecto HU-CI):* Humanizing
       Intensive Care Project, 2020, https://proyectohuci.com/en
       /home/.

182   *ICU patients get less than one hour of good sleep per day:* P. L. Wat-
       son, P. Pandharipande, B. K. Gehlbach, et al., "Atypical Sleep in
       Ventilated Patients: Empirical Electroencephalography Findings
       and the Path toward Revised ICU Sleep Scoring Criteria," *Criti-
       cal Care Medicine* 41 (2013): 1958–67.

183   *brain clears out toxins through the glymphatic system:* M. K. Rasmus-
       sen, H. Mestre, and M. Nedergaard, "The Glymphatic Pathway in
       Neurological Disorders," *Lancet Neurology* 17 (2018): 1016–24.

183   *may not activate fully in the human brain until specific stages of the
       sleep cycle:* A. R. Mendelsohn and J. W. Larrick, "Sleep Facilitates
       Clearance of Metabolites from the Brain: Glymphatic Func-
       tion in Aging and Neurodegenerative Diseases," *Rejuvenation
       Research* 16 (2013): 518–23; and H. Benveniste, P. M. Heerdt,
       M. Fontes, et al., "Glymphatic System Function in Relation to
       Anesthesia and Sleep States," *Anesthesia & Analgesia* 128 (2019):
       747–58.

183   *short sleep times may reduce the effectiveness of our brain's "waste dis-
       posal" pathway:* S. Sabia, A. Fayosse, J. Dumurgier, et al., "Asso-
       ciation of Sleep Duration in Middle and Old Age with Incidence
       of Dementia," *Nature Communications* 12 (2021): 2289, https://
       doi.org/10.1038/s41467-021-22354-2.

183   *some evidence that sedation and anesthesia impair glymphatic
       flow as well:* C. Gakuba, T. Gaberel, S. Goursaud, et al.,
       "General Anesthesia Inhibits the Activity of the 'Glymphatic
       System,'" *Theranostics* 8 (2018): 710–22.

183   *ICU sleep protocols or "nap times" are being devised and studied:*
M. P. Knauert, E. J. Gilmore, T. E. Murphy, et al., "Association
between Death and Loss of Stage N2 Sleep Features among Criti-
cally Ill Patients with Delirium," *Journal of Critical Care* 48 (2018):
124–29; M. P. Knauert, M. Pisani, N. Redeker, et al., "Pilot Study:
An Intensive Care Unit Sleep Promotion Protocol," *BMJ Open
Respiratory Research* 6 (2019): e000411; and M. P. Knauert, N. S.
Redeker, H. K. Yaggi, et al., "Creating Naptime: An Overnight,
Nonpharmacologic Intensive Care Unit Sleep Promotion Protocol," *Journal of Patient Experience* 5 (2018): 180–87.

183   *healing energy of music into our ICUs:* J. Messika, Y. Martin,
N. Maquigneau, et al., "A Musical Intervention for Respiratory
Comfort during Noninvasive Ventilation in the ICU," *European
Respiratory Journal* 53, no. 1 (2019); and L. L. Chlan, C. R.
Weinert, A. Heiderscheit, et al., "Effects of Patient-Directed
Music Intervention on Anxiety and Sedative Exposure in Criti-
cally Ill Patients Receiving Mechanical Ventilatory Support: A
Randomized Clinical Trial," *JAMA* 309 (2013): 2335–44.

184   *Dr. Carl Bäckman, a Swedish PhD nurse, first published an intrigu-
ing idea:* C. G. Bäckman and S. M. Walther, "Use of a Personal
Diary Written on the ICU during Critical Illness," *Intensive Care
Medicine* 27 (2001): 426–29.

184   *diaries worked to reduce the development of PTSD:* C. Jones,
C. Backman, M. Capuzzo, et al., "Intensive Care Diaries Reduce
New Onset Post Traumatic Stress Disorder following Critical Ill-
ness: A Randomised, Controlled Trial," *Critical Care* 14 (2010):
R168; and C. Jones, C. Bäckman, and R. D. Griffiths, "Intensive
Care Diaries and Relatives' Symptoms of Posttraumatic Stress
Disorder after Critical Illness: A Pilot Study," *American Journal of
Critical Care* 21 (2012): 172–76.

186   *Dr. Heidi Smith, a fierce advocate of the A2F bundle:* H. A. Smith,
J. Boyd, D. C. Fuchs, et al., "Diagnosing Delirium in Critically

Ill Children: Validity and Reliability of the Pediatric Confusion Assessment Method for the Intensive Care Unit," *Critical Care Medicine* 39 (2011): 150–57; and H. A. Smith, M. Gangopadhyay, C. M. Goben, et al., "The Preschool Confusion Assessment Method for the ICU: Valid and Reliable Delirium Monitoring for Critically Ill Infants and Children," *Critical Care Medicine* 44 (2016): 592–600.

188   *The Lansing family has PICS-F:* Davidson, Jones, and Bienvenu, "Family Response to Critical Illness: Postintensive Care Syndrome—Family."

188   *launch the ICU Recovery Center:* CIBS ICU Recovery Center, 2020, https://www.icudelirium.org/the-icu-recovery-center-at-vanderbilt.

188   *her interprofessional team began seeing survivors from our ICUs:* C. M. Sevin, S. L. Bloom, J. C. Jackson, et al., "Comprehensive Care of ICU Survivors: Development and Implementation of an ICU Recovery Center," *Journal of Critical Care* 46 (2018): 141–48; and C. M. Sevin and J. C. Jackson, "Post-ICU Clinics Should Be Staffed by ICU Clinicians," *Critical Care Medicine* 47 (2019): 268–72.

189   *Society of Critical Care Medicine's THRIVE Initiative:* K. J. Haines, J. McPeake, E. Hibbert, et al., "Enablers and Barriers to Implementing ICU Follow-Up Clinics and Peer Support Groups following Critical Illness: The Thrive Collaboratives," *Critical Care Medicine* 47 (2019): 1194–200; K. J. Haines, C. M. Sevin, E. Hibbert, et al., "Key Mechanisms by Which Post-ICU Activities Can Improve In-ICU Care: Results of the International THRIVE Collaboratives," *Intensive Care Medicine* 45 (2019): 939–47; and M. E. Mikkelsen, M. Still, B. J. Anderson, et al., "Society of Critical Care Medicine's International Consensus Conference on Prediction and Identification of Long-Term Impairments after Critical Illness," *Critical Care Medicine* 48, no. 11 (2020): 1670–79.

190   *These survivors, numbering in the tens of millions:* A. Nalbandian,
        K. Sehgal, and E. Y. Wan, "Post-Acute COVID-19 Syndrome,"
        Nature Medicine (2021).

193   *she founded the ARDS Foundation:* ARDS Foundation, 2020,
        https://ardsglobal.org/.

193   *narrative medicine, a relatively new field . . . Rita Charon, one of
        the field's pioneers:* R. Charon, "Narrative Medicine: A Model for
        Empathy, Reflection, Profession, and Trust," *JAMA* 286 (2001):
        1897–902; and R. Charon, *Narrative Medicine: Honoring the
        Stories of Illness* (Oxford University Press, 2008).

194   *possibilities for narrative and reflective writing to humanize:*
        H. S. Wald, "In the Here and Now," *JAMA* 299 (2008): 613–
        14; and H. S. Wald, "Optimizing Resilience and Wellbeing for
        Healthcare Professions Trainees and Healthcare Professionals
        during Public Health Crises—Practical Tips for an 'Integrative
        Resilience' Approach," *Medical Teacher* 42 (2020): 744–55.

197   *when Kaas, Merzenich, and Taub temporarily restricted the use:*
        E. Taub, G. Uswatte, V. W. Mark, et al., "The Learned Nonuse
        Phenomenon: Implications for Rehabilitation," *Europa Medico-
        physica* 42 (2006): 241–56.

197   *The brains of these animals exhibited unequivocal neuroplasticity:*
        M. Merzenich, B. Wright, W. Jenkins, et al., "Cortical Plasticity
        Underlying Perceptual, Motor, and Cognitive Skill Development:
        Implications for Neurorehabilitation," *Cold Spring Harbor Sympo-
        sia on Quantitative Biology* 61 (1996): 1–8; and M. M. Merzenich
        and R. C. deCharms, "Neural Representations, Experience, and
        Change," in *The Mind-Brain Continuum: Sensory Processes*, ed. R. R.
        Llinás and P. S. Churchland (MIT Press, 1996), 61–81.

197   *Dr. Norman Doidge's book:* N. Doidge, *The Brain That Changes
        Itself: Stories of Personal Triumph from the Frontiers of Brain Sci-
        ence* (Penguin, 2007).

197   *constraint-induced therapy (CIT):* E. Taub, V. W. Mark, and
          G. Uswatte, "Implications of CI Therapy for Visual Deficit
          Training," *Frontiers in Integrative Neuroscience* 8 (2014): 78;
          E. Taub, G. Uswatte, and V. W. Mark, "The Functional Signifi-
          cance of Cortical Reorganization and the Parallel Development
          of CI Therapy," *Frontiers in Human Neuroscience* 8 (2014): 396;
          and "Constraint-Induced Therapy (CI Therapy)," Taub Therapy
          Clinic, UAB Medicine, 2020, https://www.uabmedicine.org
          /patient-care/treatments/ci-therapy.

198   *Goal Management Training (GMT), developed by Dr. Brian Levine:*
          B. Levine, I. H. Robertson, L. Clare, et al., "Rehabilitation of Ex-
          ecutive Functioning: An Experimental-Clinical Validation of Goal
          Management Training," *Journal of the International Neuropsycho-
          logical Society* 6 (2000): 299–312; and B. Levine, T. A. Schweizer,
          C. O'Connor, et al., "Rehabilitation of Executive Functioning in
          Patients with Frontal Lobe Brain Damage with Goal Management
          Training," *Frontiers in Human Neuroscience* 5 (2011): 9.

198   *Dr. Michael Merzenich's BrainHQ cognitive exercises:* J. E. Wilson,
          E. M. Collar, A. L. Kiehl, et al., "Computerized Cognitive Reha-
          bilitation in Intensive Care Unit Survivors: Returning to Everyday
          Tasks Using Rehabilitation Networks—Computerized Cognitive
          Rehabilitation Pilot Investigation," *Annals of the American Thoracic
          Society* 15 (2018): 887–91.

198   *Dr. Adam Gazzaley, from the University of California, San Fran-
          cisco:* J. A. Anguera, J. Boccanfuso, J. L. Rintoul, et al., "Video
          Game Training Enhances Cognitive Control in Older Adults,"
          Nature 501 (2013): 97–101; and A. S. Berry, T. P. Zanto, W. C.
          Clapp, et al., "The Influence of Perceptual Training on Working
          Memory in Older Adults," *PLoS One* 5 (2010): e11537.

199   *determining the exact nature of acquired dementia after critical illness:*
          "Alzheimer's Disease & Related Dementias (ADRD)," NIH, 2020,
          https://www.nia.nih.gov/health/alzheimers; and "NIA-Funded

Active Alzheimer's and Related Dementias Clinical Trials and Studies," https://www.nia.nih.gov/research/ongoing-AD-trials.

199   *BRAIN-2 study:* "The BRAIN-2 Study," Grantome, 2020, https://grantome.com/grant/NIH/R01-AG058639-01A1.

200   *they studied the gray matter volume in the hippocampus:* E. A. Maguire, D. G. Gadian, I. S. Johnsrude, et al., "Navigation-Related Structural Change in the Hippocampi of Taxi Drivers," *Proceedings of the National Academy of Sciences* 97 (2000): 4398–403; E. A. Maguire, K. Woollett, and H. J. Spiers, "London Taxi Drivers and Bus Drivers: A Structural MRI and Neuropsychological Analysis," *Hippocampus* 16 (2006): 1091–101; and K. Woollett and E. A. Maguire, "Acquiring 'the Knowledge' of London's Layout Drives Structural Brain Changes," *Current Biology* 21 (2011): 2109–14.

202   *mechanically ventilated patients lose nearly 20 percent:* Z. A. Puthucheary, J. Rawal, M. McPhail, et al., "Acute Skeletal Muscle Wasting in Critical Illness," *JAMA* 310 (2013): 1591–600.

202   *they can rapidly age into frailty:* N. E. Brummel, T. D. Girard, P. P. Pandharipande, et al., "Prevalence and Course of Frailty in Survivors of Critical Illness," *Critical Care Medicine* 48 (2020): 1419–26; and K. Rockwood, X. Song, C. MacKnight, et al., "A Global Clinical Measure of Fitness and Frailty in Elderly People," *Canadian Medical Association Journal* 173 (2005): 489–95.

203   *fifty-two studies of over ten thousand previously employed ICU survivors:* Kamdar et al., "Return to Work after Critical Illness: A Systematic Review and Meta-Analysis."

203   *These figures and those from other studies:* Norman et al., "Employment Outcomes After Critical Illness"; B. B. Kamdar, M. Huang,

V. D. Dinglas, et al., "Joblessness and Lost Earnings after Acute Respiratory Distress Syndrome in a 1-Year National Multicenter Study," *American Journal of Respiratory and Critical Care Medicine* 196 (2017): 1012–20; and J. McPeake, M. E. Mikkelsen, T. Quasim, et al., "Return to Employment after Critical Illness and Its Association with Psychosocial Outcomes. A Systematic Review and Meta-Analysis," *Annals of the American Thoracic Society* 16 (2019): 1304–11.

205   *Vanderbilt colleague Dr. Jonathan Metzl's work:* J. M. Metzl and H. Hansen, "Structural Competency: Theorizing a New Medical Engagement with Stigma and Inequality," *Social Science & Medicine* 103 (2014): 126–33; and J. M. Metzl, A. Maybank, and F. De Maio, "Responding to the COVID-19 Pandemic: The Need for a Structurally Competent Health Care System," *JAMA* 324, no 3. (2020): 231–32.

205   *Epigenetics research . . . demonstrates that high-stress, resource-poor conditions can create risk:* S. E. Johnstone and S. B. Baylin, "Stress and the Epigenetic Landscape: A Link to the Pathobiology of Human Diseases?," *Nature Reviews Genetics* 11 (2010): 806–12.

206   *Neuroscientists have found that social exclusion, poverty, and chronic stress:* G. W. Evans and M. A. Schamberg, "Childhood Poverty, Chronic Stress, and Adult Working Memory," *Proceedings of the National Academy of Sciences* 106 (2009): 6545–49; and B. Buwalda, M. H. Kole, A. H. Veenema, et al., "Long-Term Effects of Social Stress on Brain and Behavior: A Focus on Hippocampal Functioning," *Neuroscience & Biobehavioral Reviews* 29 (2005): 83–97.

206   *economists have shown that when people with low income:* J. Ludwig, L. Sanbonmatsu, L. Gennetian, et al., "Neighborhoods, Obesity, and Diabetes—A Randomized Social Experiment," *New England Journal of Medicine* 365 (2011): 1509–19.

Chapter 12: End-of-Life Care in the ICU—Patient and Family Wishes Can Come True

210 *One in five deaths in the United States occurs in a critical care bed:*
D. C. Angus, A. E. Barnato, W. T. Linde-Zwirble, et al., "Use of
Intensive Care at the End of Life in the United States: An Epide-
miologic Study," *Critical Care Medicine* 32 (2004): 638–43.

217 *body of studies and scientific literature about letting people go:* C. S.
Hartog, D. Schwarzkopf, C. L. Sprung, et al., "End-of-Life Care
in the Intensive Care Unit: A Patient-Based Questionnaire of
Intensive Care Unit Staff Perception and Relatives' Psychologi-
cal Response," *Palliative Medicine* 29, no. 4 (2021): 336–45;
P. Jabre, V. Belpomme, E. Azoulay, et al., "Family Presence
During Cardiopulmonary Resuscitation," *New England Journal
of Medicine* 368, no. 11 (2013): 1008–18; J. R. Curtis, D. L.
Patrick, I. Byock, et al., "A Measure of the Quality of Dying
and Death. Initial Validation Using After-Death Interviews with
Family Members," *Journal of Pain and Symptom Management* 24,
no. 1 (2002): 17–31; J. N. Zitter, *Extreme Measures: Finding a
Better Path to the End of Life* (Avery, 2017); I. Byock, *Dying Well:
Peace and Possibilities at the End of Life* (Riverhead Books, 1998);
D. B. White, D. C. Angus, A. M. Shields, et al., "A Randomized
Trial of a Family-Support Intervention in Intensive Care Units,"
New England Journal of Medicine 378, no. 25 (2018): 2365–75.

218 *Deborah's 3 Wishes Project helps physicians and family members:*
D. Cook, M. Swinton, F. Toledo, et al., "Personalizing Death in
the Intensive Care Unit: The 3 Wishes Project: A Mixed-Methods
Study," *Annals of Internal Medicine* 163 (2015): 271–79.

222 Elderhood, *geriatrician Dr. Louise Aronson highlights the negative
effects:* L. Aronson, *Elderhood: Redefining Aging, Transforming Medicine, Reimagining Life* (Bloomsbury Publishing USA,
2019).

224   *report released by the National Academy of Medicine:* National Academy of Medicine, *Taking Action against Clinician Burnout: A Systems Approach to Professional Well-Being* (National Academies Press, 2019).

224   *and this was before the COVID-19 pandemic:* N. Kok, J. van Gurp, S. Teerenstra, et al., "Coronavirus Disease 2019 Immediately Increases Burnout Symptoms in ICU Professionals: A Longitudinal Cohort Study," *Critical Care Medicine* 49 (2021): 419–27.

225   JAMA *paper, Dr. Donna Zulman and author-physician Dr. Abraham Verghese:* D. M. Zulman, M. C. Haverfield, J. G. Shaw, et al., "Practices to Foster Physician Presence and Connection with Patients in the Clinical Encounter," *JAMA* 323 (2020): 70–81.

226   *As Drs. Stephen Trzeciak and Anthony Mazzarelli state:* S. Trzeciak and A. Mazzarelli, *Compassionomics: The Revolutionary Scientific Evidence That Caring Makes a Difference* (Studer Group, 2019).

227   *three out of four hospitalized patients prefer that their physician ask about:* C. K. Alch, K. M. Collier, and R. Y. Yeow, "Addressing Spiritual and Religious Needs in Advanced Illness: A Teachable Moment," *JAMA Internal Medicine* 181, no. 1 (2021): 115–16; D. E. King and B. Bushwick, "Beliefs and Attitudes of Hospital Inpatients about Faith Healing and Prayer," *Journal of Family Practice* 39 (1994): 349–52; C. D. MacLean, B. Susi, N. Phifer, et al., "Patient Preference for Physician Discussion and Practice of Spirituality," *Journal of General Internal Medicine* 18 (2003): 38–43; D. P. Sulmasy, "Spirituality, Religion, and Clinical Care," *Chest* 135 (2009): 1634–42; R. J. Wall, R. A. Engelberg, C. J. Gries, et al., "Spiritual Care of Families in the Intensive Care Unit," *Critical Care Medicine* 35 (2007): 1084–90; B. Lo, D. Ruston, L. W. Kates, et al., "Discussing Religious and Spiritual Issues at the End of Life: A Practical Guide for Physicians," *JAMA* 287 (2002): 749–54; K. E. Steinhauser, C. I. Voils, E. C.

Clipp, et al., "'Are You at Peace?': One Item to Probe Spiritual Concerns at the End of Life," *Archives of Internal Medicine* 166 (2006): 101–5; J. W. Ehman, B. B. Ott, T. H. Short, et al., "Do Patients Want Physicians to Inquire about Their Spiritual or Religious Beliefs If They Become Gravely Ill?," *Archives of Internal Medicine* 159 (1999): 1803–6; and K. M. Collier, C. A. James, S. Saint, et al., "Is It Time to More Fully Address Teaching Religion and Spirituality in Medicine?," *Annals of Internal Medicine* 172 (2020): 817–18.

229   *Pope Benedict XVI, was asked:* J. Ratzinger, *Salt of the Earth: The Church at the End of the Millennium* (Ignatius Press, 1996).

Epilogue

235   *we studied more than two thousand COVID-ICU patients:* B. T. Pun et al., "Prevalence and Risk Factors for Delirium in Critically Ill Patients with COVID-19 (COVID-D): A Multicentre Cohort Study."

236   *"I'm sticking to the A2F bundle":* D. R. Janz, S. Mackey, N. Patel, et al., "Critically Ill Adults with Coronavirus Disease 2019 in New Orleans and Care with an Evidence-Based Protocol," *Chest* 159 (January 2021): 196–204.

237   *In* Being Mortal, *Dr. Atul Gawande outlines the stark reality:* A. Gawande, *Being Mortal: Medicine and What Matters in the End* (Metropolitan Books, 2014), 18.

237   *I have a practice whereby:* E. W. Ely, "Each Person Is a World in COVID-19," *Lancet* (January 22, 2021).

239   *Dietrich Bonhoeffer in a letter he wrote:* D. Bonhoeffer, *Letters and Papers from Prison* (Fortress Press, 2010).

242   *I was in Zambia studying delirium:* J. K. Banerdt, K. Mateyo, L. Wang, et al., "Delirium as a Predictor of Mortality and Disability

Among Hospitalized Patients in Zambia," *PLoS One* 16 (February 11, 2021): e0246330.

243   *Carla Davis, who leads Heart of Hospice:* H. Vossel, "Heart of Hospice's Carla Davis: Rise to the COVID-19 Challenge," Hospice News, April 3, 2020, https://hospicenews.com/2020/04/03 /heart-of-hospices-carla-davis-rise-to-the-covid-19%EF%BB%BF -challenge/; and "Carla Davis," Heart of Hospice, 2020, https:// www.heartofhospice.net/agency-staff/carla-davis.

PERMISSIONS

GRATEFUL ACKNOWLEDGMENT IS MADE for permission to reprint the following:

• • •

• • •

Index

AARP, 272n, 273n, 274

ABC trial, 118, 121–23, 127–29, 135, 168

ABCDEF (A2F) bundle, 168, 171, 172, 255–56

Acosta, Dr. Lealani, 156–57, 159, 160, 161

acute respiratory distress syndrome (ARDS), 52–53, 193, 274
  COVID with, 222, 244
  ICU experience of, 19, 135, 177, 206–7
  long-term impact of, 138

Adams, Kelly McCutcheon, 166, 170

"Aequanimitas" (Osler), 70

aging, 80, 93, 272

aging brain, myths about, 272–73

Akili, 198

Al-Anon, 229

alveoli, 51, 52

Alzheimer's Disease and Related Dementias (ADRDs), 199.
  See also dementia

American Thoracic Society, 258

analgesia, 168, 255, 257

Andersen, Hans Christian, 136, 154

Andersen, Dr. Poul Klint, 140

anesthesia
  assessment of reactions to, 121
  brain impact of, 183
  early overdosing of, 120–21
  ideal sedation depth for, 126

anesthesiologists, delirium tips for, 257

Angelou, Maya, 4, 41–43, 57, 207–8

Angus, Dr. Derek, 32

antipsychotics, 56, 79, 131, 160, 175, 257

anxiety
  caregivers' risk for, 262
  family members with, 25, 187, 222
  ICU experience of, 23, 25, 94, 160, 191
  ICU survivors' risk for, 25
  medications for, 8, 130, 135, 210
  music in ICUs to lessen, 183
  PICS and, 138, 259
  sedation for, 8, 130, 135, 234
  treatment for, 201, 261, 269

Appleby, Dr. Scott, 221

ARDS. See acute respiratory distress syndrome

ARDS Foundation, 193

Aristotle, 70

Armstrong, Louis, 52

Aronson, Dr. Louise, 222
Arrowsmith (Lewis), 107
astrocytes, 200
atheist, 227, 228
attention and concentration difficulties
  delirium and, 84, 85, 90, 204, 248,
    249
  ICU survivors and, 20, 89, 204
  resources for, 268
A2F (ABCDEF) bundle, 168, 171,
  172, 255–56
Awakenings (Sacks), 103, 142
Awdish, Rana, 95
Azoulay, Dr. Élie, 217

Bäckman, Dr. Carl, 184
Bailey, Polly, 139, 144–46, 153, 154,
  168, 215
Balas, Dr. Michele, 173
Balser, Dr. Jeff, 107
Barnes-Daly, Mary Ann "Jett," 171,
  172, 175
Barnes-Jewish Hospital, St. Louis,
  Missouri, 58, 60, 65, 67
Bastarache, Dr. Julie, 174
behavior
  addictions and, 229
  brain injuries reflected in, 84
  cognitive difficulties and changes
    in, 270
  delirium shown through, 78, 248
  epigenetics research on, 205
  malignant normality of, 131
  mobility and, 154
Being Mortal (Gawande), 237
Bellow, Saul, 119

beneficence, xi, 104
benevolence, xi, 83, 104
benzodiazepines
  brain monitoring of action of,
    126–27
  delirium prevention by avoiding,
    257
  ICU dependence on, 124
  ICU high doses of, 8, 55, 131, 160,
    162
  PICS and, 263
  as predictor of delirium, 162–63,
    236
  sleep problems from, 182
  randomized controlled trials, 118,
    127–29
Bernard, Dr. Claude, 39
Bernard, Dr. Gordon, 123
Berwick, Dr. Donald, 166, 167, 170
Betters, Dr. Kristina, 186, 188
Billian, Carol (patient), 194–95, 200
bioethics, 116, 217, 218
BiPAP breathing mask, 213, 230, 289
bispectral index (BIS) in brain
  monitoring, 126, 127
Bjørneboe, Dr. Mogens, 35–36, 37
bleeding, 109, 234, 279
Blegdams Hospital, Denmark, 35–38
Blink (Gladwell), 196
blood, 1, 96, 209
  clots in, 128, 151
  CPR and, 6
  displaced femur fracture and, 214
  draws of, 2, 7, 8, 46, 104, 187, 239
  ECMO processing of, 28, 186
  feet swelling with, 223

hemophagocytic
   lymphohistiocytosis (HLH) and,
   231
H1N1 influenza's impact on, 23
investigations using, xii
kidney dialysis of, 7
lab analysis of, 9, 46, 204, 271
lymphatic system and, 182–83
medications in, 131
oxygen levels in, 63
transfusions of, 110, 232
tumors and, 120
blood banks, 38
Blood on the Tracks (Dylan), 282
blood vessels, 51, 63, 68, 90, 120, 214
Bollich, Sarah (patient), 55
Bonhoeffer, Dietrich, 239
Bowlin, Todd (patient), 202–3
brain
   astrocytes in, 200
   boosting health of, 22, 273–74
   chronic traumatic encephalopathy
      (CTE) and, 161
   glial cells in, 199–200, 201
   impact of sedation and anesthesia
      on, 183
   Lewy body dementia and, 199
   memory and, 97, 109, 158
   microglia in, 200
   myths about aging in, 272–73
   neurogenesis and, 201, 272
   synapses in, 199–200
   synaptogenesis in, 201
   System 1 and System 2 thinking in,
      196, 198–99
brain fog, 89, 190, 253

brain HQ cognitive exercises, 198, 267
brain injury, and delirium, 84, 90, 112
brain monitoring, in sedation, 126,
   127
brain problems, after ICU discharge,
   14–15, 17. *See also* post-intensive
   care syndrome (PICS)
Brain That Changes Itself, The
   (Doidge), 197
breathing
   BiPAP masks for help in, 213, 230,
      289
   COVID-19 patient's description of,
      244
   decision to remove ventilators and,
      66, 81
   diagnostic tests of, 119
   observing in physical exam, 41
   polio's impact on, 35
   setting up ventilators for, 52
breathing problems
   COVID and, 28–30
   ICU monitors of respiratory
      function in, 51–52
   inverse ratio ventilation (IRV) in,
      53–54
   lung function and, 50–51
   PEEP readings in, 52–53
   subcutaneous emphysema and,
      29–30
   ventilator innovation during polio
      epidemics and, 34–37, 50, 133
Buber, Martin, 69, 70
bundle (ICU protocol), *see* A2F
   (ABCDEF) bundle, 168
Byock, Dr. Ira, 217

cancer, 59, 72–73, 213, 217
caregivers
  organ transplantation and, 60
  patients' stories of their critical
    illnesses and, 207
  PICS and, 262
  quality of life for, 87
  resources for, 247–54
Cassem, Dr. Edwin "Ned," 78
Chanute, Octave, 155
Charity Hospital, New Orleans, 2–3,
  33, 65, 236, 242
Charon, Dr. Rita, 194
chest tubes, 8, 28, 193
chest X-rays, 29, 115, 119, 180
childbirth
  peripartum cardiomyopathy after, 5–6
  treatments creating harm after, 151
children, ARDS in, 53
Chin, Dr. Bob, 46–47, 48
choice of drug, 168, 255
chronic traumatic encephalopathy
  (CTE), 161
CIBS Center, Vanderbilt University
  and VA Medical Center, Nashville
  ICU Recovery Center at, 188–89,
    193
  multifold approach to PICS at,
    198–99
  resources from, 247
  support sessions at, 16–17, 86–88,
    247
Clemmer, Dr. Terry, 145–46, 168
Clinical Frailty Scale, 202
clinical trials, 83, 110, 111, 141, 142,
  255

ABC trial, 118, 121–23, 127–29,
  135, 168
  brain HQ cognitive exercises used
    in, 198
  of ICU diaries, 184
  MENDS trial, 118, 123–25, 129
Cobb, Marcus (patient), 63–65,
  67–69, 70–71
cognitive impairment
  after ICU delirium, 92, 104, 105–6,
    108–9
  delirium risk related to, 250
  life-support removal and, 127, 140
  screening for, 251, 257
cognitive rehabilitation, 198, 201,
  267–70
cohort studies, 255
Common Sense (Paine), 75
compassion, xii, 95, 143–44, 179,
  207, 219, 225, 226, 238, 243,
  245
Compassionomics (Trzeciak and
  Mazzarelli), 226
compliance, 171, 172, 173, 175, 198,
  206
confusion. See also delirium
  ICU conditions and, 181
  patients' experiences of, 19, 56, 76,
    78, 90, 161
  patients' self-awareness of, 248
  as possible symptom of delirium,
    79, 249
Confusion Assessment Method for the
  ICU (CAM-ICU), 84–85, 86, 160
constraint-induced therapy (CIT),
  197–98

Cook, Dr. Deborah, 86, 126–27, 140, 218–19
Correa, Victor, 209–11, 212
COVID-19
 cost of survival of, 16
 delirium and, 76, 94
 extracorporeal membrane oxygenation (ECMO) for, 28
 ICU unit for, 28–30
 patient's experience of, 75–76
 PICS risk and, 262–63
 subcutaneous emphysema in, 29–30
 See also Long COVID
critical care
 ABCDEF (A2F) bundle, 168, 171, 172, 255–56
 criticism of sedation and paralysis approach in, 57–58
 delirium reported by patients in, 81–82
 discharged patients on experience of, 8–10, 104–6
 helpful websites for, 274–75
 history of, 27–43
 inverse ratio ventilation (IRV) in, 53–54
 muscle atrophy in, 151, 153
 PEEP readings in, 52–53
 saving lives as goal in, 10–11, 26, 48–49
 ventilator innovation during polio epidemics and, 34–37, 50
Critical Illness, Brain Dysfunction, and Survivorship (CIBS) Center. *See* CIBS Center

culture of critical care, 10, 26, 49, 172–73, 174, 234
Cure at Troy, The (Heaney), 133
Curie, Marie, 27
Curtis, Dr. Randy, 217
Cutting for Stone (Verghese), 115
cystic fibrosis, 39–40, 61

Dahl, Ophelia, 216
daily life difficulties, resources for, 271–72
Dalai Lama, 197
Dandy, Walter, 33
Davidson, Dr. Judy, 138
Davis, Carla, 243–44
DeBakey, Dr. Michael, 2
delirium, 75–94
 assessment method (CAM-ICU) for, 84–85, 86, 160
 attention problems in, 84, 85, 90, 204, 248, 249
 brain injury and, 84, 90, 112
 brain monitoring of sedation and, 126–27
 caregivers and, 252–54
 classic medical approach to, 79–80
 cognitive impairment after, 92, 104, 105–6, 108–9
 COVID and, 76, 94
 definition of, 90–91
 determining extent of brain injury in, 199
 dexmedetomidine trial with, 123–25
 evaluating patients for, 256

delirium (*cont.*)

  family members' role in treating, 93, 257

  family's awareness of, 79, 81, 93–94, 111

  finding funding for research on causes of, 110–11, 121–22

  hallucinations with, 78, 79, 87–89, 90, 91–92, 264

  helpful websites for, 274–75

  ICU patients' experiences of, 81–82, 89, 111, 124

  ICU survivors' experience of, 111–13, 119

  intubated patients' reporting of, 84–85

  manifestations of, 90–91

  older theories of, 83–84

  physician's observation of signs of, 78–79

  as predictor of death, 103–4

  recommendations on, 256–57

  resources for understanding, 248–51

  risk-reduction strategies for, 93

  as sedation complication, 58

  screening for, 86, 251, 257

  support group stories about, 86–94

  tips for anesthesiologists and surgeons about, 257

  tips for dealing with, 251–54

dementia

  aging brain and, 272

  benzodiazepine use as predictor of, 162–63

  brain MRI research in, 158

  delirium risk related to, 250

  helpful websites for, 274–75

  ICU-acquired, 15, 157, 159, 176, 259

  ICU experiences of, 157–58, 159, 162

  impact of on ICU survivors, 191–92

  multifold cognitive rehabilitation approach to, 198

  sedation and anesthesia in ICU and, 183

Department of Veterans Affairs, 110, 198

depersonalization, xii, 69, 180, 208, 241

depression

  caregivers' risk for, 262

  COVID-19 and risk for, 224

  delirium risk related to, 250

  ICU experiences of, 23, 24, 160, 162, 191, 194, 207

  ICU survivors' risk for, 25

  PICS and, 16, 25, 138, 251, 259

  relatives of ICU survivors with, 25

  treatment of, 201, 261, 269

dexmedetomidine, 123–25

diagnosis

  consolidating person and, 70, 78, 224

  examples of, 90, 156, 187, 228, 238

  ICU deaths and, 210

  ICU treatment and, 51

dialysis, 1, 8, 23, 28, 31, 163, 170, 186, 204, 223

diaries in ICUs, 134, 184–85, 201–2, 253, 260, 264

Diary of Anne Frank, The (Frank), 183–84

Diffusion of Innovations (Rogers), 33

dignity, xi, 181, 203, 207, 220, 252

disabilities
  cognitive, 21, 160–61, 196
  helpful websites for, 274–75
  ICU-acquired, 15, 191
  PICS with, 138, 189, 259
  treatment of, 231

disability insurance, 189, 265

disparity, 206, 207

DNR (Do Not Resuscitate) order, 127, 213

Doctor, The (Fildes), 100–101

Doidge, Dr. Norman, 197

Donabedian, Dr. Avedis, 167, 178

Do Not Resuscitate (DNR) order, 127, 213

Dostoyevsky, Fyodor, 179

downstream problems, 189, 206, 235

Drew, Dr. Charles, 38–39

Drinker, Philip, 34

driving, and ICU survivors, 17, 20, 113, 119

drugs. *See also* benzodiazepines;
    sedatives and sedation; *and
    specific drugs*
  ABC trial and, 118
  anesthesia and, 120
  choice of, 168, 255
  MENDS trial and, 118
  stopping, in A2F bundle, 168, 255

Drumright, Kelly, 174

Dylan, Bob, 282

dyspnea, 210

early mobility, 137–39, 148–50

East of Eden (Steinbeck), 137, 150

Ebert, Vivi, 36, 37

Ebola, 237

Edmonson, Steve (patient), 192

Eger, Dr. Edmond "Ted," 121

Eisenmenger's syndrome, 63

Elderhood (Aronson), 222

elderly, 80–81, 122, 149, 222, 237

Ely, Dr. Kim Adams, 40, 67, 95–98, 101–2, 137–38, 239

emergency rooms, 2–3, 29–30, 96–97

empathy, xi, 137, 143–44, 146, 208, 210, 224, 225

emphysema, 29–30, 119, 135, 169

encephalopathy, 161. *See also* delirium

end-of-life care, 209–32
  decisions about, in ICU, 115–17
  factors in decision for life-support
    removal in, 126–27, 140
  in Haiti, 214–16
  ICU patients' experiences of,
    209–11, 212, 213, 220–21,
    222–23, 228–29, 231–32
  impact on doctors and nurses of,
    224–26
  palliative care and, 216–20
  spirituality of patients and, 227–29,
    230–31
  spouse's feeling of exclusion from, 117

Engel, Dr. George, 80

Engel, Heidi, 168, 173

epigenetics, 205–6

errors
  in judgment, 182
  in medications, 131

Esteban, Andrés, 66
ethics, 116–17, 164, 178, 217, 218
Eucharist, 230–31
European Society of Intensive Care
    Medicine, 128
Evers, Medgar, 59–60
every deep-drawn breath, vii, 69, 137
exercise
    brain, 195, 198–99, 200, 266
    physical, 42, 146, 148, 153, 168,
        202–3, 251, 255, 261, 266, 269,
        270, 271, 273
extracorporeal membrane oxygenation
    (ECMO), 28, 186, 222–23

faith, 230–31, 273
family members
    awareness of delirium by, 79, 81,
        93–94, 111
    delirium recommendations for,
        256–57
    delirium support by, 93, 257
    end-of-life decisions and, 209–11,
        212, 216, 221–22, 223, 228–29
    general guide to PICS for, 258–62
    ICU open visitation policy for, 101
    impact of PICS on, 262
    life of ICU survivors with, 24–25,
        144–46
    PICS detection by, 259
    support interventions for, 217
Farmer, Dr. Paul, 214, 216
fatigue, resources for managing, 271
FDA, 198
feeding tubes, 31, 91, 151
Feynman, Richard, 107

Fildes, Luke, 100–101
Finfer, Dr. Simon, 32
Finnegan, Dr. Michael, 52–53
Fitzgerald, F. Scott, 65–66
frailty, 202, 234, 269
Frank, Anne, 183–84
Frankl, Viktor, 22
Fraser, Dr. Gil, 121
Frost, Robert, 42
Fugate, Ray (patient), 75–76, 94

Gawande, Dr. Atul, 237
Gazzaley, Dr. Adam, 198
geriatric medicine, 58, 80, 93
geriatrics, 80
"Gift Outright, The" (Frost), 42
Gladwell, Malcolm, 168, 196
glial cells, 199–200, 201
Goal Management Training (GMT),
    198
Gödel, Escher, Bach (Hofstadter), 282
Gordon and Betty Moore Foundation,
    171, 173
Gororo, Lovemore (patient), 86,
    89–90, 92, 195
Grenvik, Ake, 39
Griffiths, Dr. Richard, 139, 151–54,
    193, 215
Guyton, A. C., 49, 51, 67, 83

Haiti, 214–16
Hall, Dr. Jesse, 118, 139
Hallucinations and/or delusions, in
    delirium, 78, 79, 87–89, 90,
    91–92, 264
haloperidol, 56, 78, 131, 175

Halpern, Dr. Jodi, 143–44

Haponik, Dr. Ed, 40–42, 80, 141

Hardy, Dr. James, 51

harm, xi, 10, 25–26, 76, 91, 103, 104–5, 126, 128, 129, 131–32, 145, 146–47, 151, 168, 233, 236, 255

Harmer, Bonnie, 155–57, 159–62

Harmer, Rob (patient), 155–59, 160–63

Harter, Yvonne, 124–25

Hartog, Dr. Christiane, 217

Hazzard, Dr. William, 58–59, 80

health, social determinants of, 205

health care, 2, 10–11, 30–33, 39, 91, 100, 112, 129, 163, 166, 167, 205–6, 214, 234–35

health insurance, 189–90, 265

Heaney, Seamus, 133

heart failure, 222, 250

Heart of Hospice, 243–44

Heras La Calle, Dr. Gabriel, 180, 181–82

Herridge, Dr. Margaret, 139

heterotopic ossification, 9

Hill, Lamar (patient), 192

Hill, Mary and Phillip (patients), 238–39

Hilley, Donna (patient), 111–13

Hinton, S. E., 4

Hippocrates, 83

Hippocratic oath, 40

Hirshfield, Jane, 209

HIV/AIDS, 242

Holt, Tisha (patient), 244

Hope, Dr. Aluko, 189

Hopkins, Dr. Ramona, 158

hospice, 213, 243

House of God, The (Shem), 69

humanism, 73, 174, 219

humanity, xii, 3, 10, 11, 73, 74, 100–101, 142, 167, 176, 185, 236, 242, 252

Humanizing Intensive Care project (Proyecto HU-CI), 180, 182

humanness, 207

Hunter, Clementine, 239–42

Huslid, Audun (patient), 191, 263

Hyzy, Dr. Robert, 235

Ibsen, Dr. Bjørn, 35–36, 37, 39

ICU diaries, 134, 184–85, 201–2, 253, 260, 264

ICU Liberation Collaborative, Society of Critical Care Medicine (SCCM), 173–74, 175, 255

ICU patients
anesthesia assessment in, 121
delirium reported by, 81–82, 86–91
dementia acquired by. See dementia
diaries used by, 134, 184–85, 201–2, 253, 260, 264
early mobility and walking by, 137–39, 148–50
muscle atrophy in, 151, 153
physical therapists' work with, 136, 139, 146, 147–48, 165, 174, 186
reduction in likelihood of death for over thirty-year period, 32
sedation used with. See sedatives and sedation
spouse's feeling of exclusion from care of, 117

ICU psychosis, 56, 79, 112, 131. *See also* delirium

ICU Recovery Center, Vanderbilt University Medical Center, Nashville, 188–89, 193

ICUs (intensive care units), 30–32
cost per square foot to build, 30–31
family's experience of treatment in, 99–100
ICU psychosis as side effect in, 56, 79, 112, 131
innovation medical technology and, 39–40
life of patients after discharge from. *See* ICU survivors
number of beds in, compared with overall hospital beds, 31
number of hospitals with, 31–32
open family visitation policy in, 101
patients in. *See* ICU patients
problems after discharge from, 14–15. *See also* post-intensive care syndrome (PICS)
reduction in likelihood of death in, 32
saving lives as only goal in, 48–49
"sedate and immobilize" standard in, 45–56
sepsis as leading reason for admission to, 32

ICU survivors
attention difficulties in, 20, 89, 204
brain and body problems of, 14–15. *See also* post-intensive care syndrome (PICS)
percentage of developing problems after ICU discharge, 16

physical therapists' work with, 202–3, 265

PICS and. *See* post-intensive care syndrome (PICS)
psychological changes in, 24–25
support groups for. *See* support groups for ICU survivors

Idiot, The (Dostoyevsky), 179

Ignatius of Loyola, 69

I Know Why the Caged Bird Sings (Angelou), 4, 41, 57

infection, 54
as complication of ICU stay, 58, 128
COVID and, xii, 190, 206, 237, 262, 263
delirium and, 250, 256
HIV and, 242
lung, 14, 42, 61
patients' experiences of, 14, 48, 158, 176–77, 193
PICS and, 259–60
sepsis and, 32, 39, 54
transplantation and risk for, 61, 62

injustice, 4, 60, 117, 174, 205

innovation, 33–40
background to theory of, 33–34
critical care changes from, 38–40
early adopters in, 33–34
early mobility in ICU and, 144
physician's goal of saving lives and, 40
shift in thinking in medical community and, 37, 40
transplant medicine and, 59
ventilator innovation during polio epidemics example of, 34–37, 50

Inouye, Dr. Sharon, 84, 93
In Shock (Awdish), 95
Institute for Healthcare Improvement
(IHI), 166, 167, 170, 173
intelligence (IQ) testing, 20–21
intensive care delirium, 58. *See also*
delirium
Intensive Care Delirium Screening
Checklist, 86
intensive care units. *See* ICU *entries*
intensivist doctors, 17, 28, 53, 134,
138, 180, 185, 186, 188, 195,
234
intubated patients
communication between nurses and,
135–36, 147
research assessment of delirium in,
84–85
intubation in ICUs
example of emergency use of, 45–47
inverse ratio ventilation (IRV), 53–54
iron lungs, 34–35, 36
isolation, xii, 25, 164, 211, 222, 263
Iwashyna, Dr. Jack, 189

Jackson, Dr. James "Jim," 17, 18, 19,
20–21, 108, 158, 247
Jefferson, Dr. Angela, 199
Jepsen, Dr. Søren, 140
Jirut, Dr. Paisal (patient), 228
Johns Hopkins Hospital, 33, 138
Johnson, Guy, 207–8
Johnson, Jimmie (patient), 220–21
Jones, Dr. Christina, 134, 184, 193,
201–2
Journal of the American Medical

Association (*JAMA*), 86, 129, 144,
171, 225
Journal of Neuropsychiatry, 79–80

Kaas, Dr. Jon, 196, 197
Kahneman, Dr. Daniel, 196
Kalanithi, Paul, 13
Kandel, Dr. Eric, 83, 97
Keenan, James F., 143
Keener, Susan (patient), 222–23
Keith, Janet (patient), 86, 176–78
kidney failure, 7, 19, 29, 177, 186
Kim, Yu-hyun (patient), 234
Knauert, Dr. Melissa, 183
Knowles, John, 4
Kress, Dr. J. P., 118, 139

Laënnec, Dr. René, 62
Lancet, 133, 141, 168, 171
Langford, Richard (patient), 13–16,
17–18, 25, 26, 86, 158
Lansing, Titus (patient), 186–88
Lassen, Dr. Henry, 35–36
Lassen-Greene, Dr. Caroline, 87, 247
Leaves of Grass (Whitman), 233
Levine, Dr. Brian, 198
Lewis, Sinclair, 107
Lewy body dementia, 199
life support, 7, 19, 69, 77, 163, 173,
177, 245
advocates needed for patients on,
101
cost of, 31
decision for removal of, 66, 116,
126–27, 140
delirium dreams during, 24

life support (*cont.*)
  machines used for, 41, 50
  patients' reactions to, 78, 194
  sedation during, 78, 120
Lifton, Robert Jay, 131
loneliness, 105, 181, 207, 222
lonely feelings, 82
Long COVID, 190, 262, 263
long-haulers, 190, 262
lung cancer, 59, 72–73
lung problems. *See* breathing problems
lung transplantation, first surgery for,
  59–60. *See also* transplantation

Maclean, Norman, 1, 166–67
Maguire, Dr. Eleanor, 200–201
malignant normality, 131
Mandela, Nelson, 233
Man's Search for Meaning (Frankl), 22
Marshall, Dr. John, 32
Martin, Teresa (patient), 7–10, 15, 48,
  58, 112, 130–31, 245–46
Massachusetts General Hospital, 33,
  35, 120
Matas, Dr. Rudolph, 2
Mateyo, Dr. Kondwelani, 242–43
Maze, Dr. Mervyn, 124, 125, 129
Mazzarelli, Dr. Anthony, 226
medical team members
  evaluating for delirium by, 256
  recommendations about delirium
    from, 256–57
  resources for, 255–57
medications. *See also* benzodiazepines;
  sedatives and sedation; *and*
  specific medications

anesthesia and, 121, 257
choice of, 168, 255
critical care and, 31
delirium and, 250, 252, 256, 257
discharge planning for, 264–65
dose response to, 175
fatigue management with, 271
hospitalization preparation with list
  of, 251, 254
ICU sleep disruptions from, 182
ICU survivors' confusion about, 14,
  105, 158
life support with, 7
lung transplants and, 62, 68–69
managing, 268
memory impairment and, 267
pain control and, 257
personal needs in setting schedules
  for, 182, 189, 212
PICS and, 26, 261
potential harm from, 104, 131
sepsis and, 32
sleep and, 271
ventilated patients and, 78, 260
medicine
  classic approach to delirium in,
    79–80
  desire for more humanity in, 73–74
  innovation in, 33–40
  reaction to overreliance on science
    by, 100–101
  seeing the patient as a whole person
    in, 69–71
  shift in thinking about life-saving
    technology in, 37, 40
Melton, Mike (patient), 228–29

memory, and brain functions, 97, 109, 158

memory impairment
cognitive therapy for, 203, 267, 272
delirium and, 249
ICU survivors with, 112, 119, 158, 191, 249
mood symptoms and, 269
resources for, 267–68
See also dementia

MENDS trial, 118, 123–25, 129

mental health issues
follow-up post-ICU treatment of, 188, 189, 201, 261
ICU stay related to, 159–60
PICS and, 15–16, 138, 259

mercy, 143

Merzenich, Dr. Michael, 196, 197, 198

Metzl, Dr. Jonathan, 205

microglia, 200

Miller, Sarah Beth (patient), 17–22, 25, 26, 86, 87–89, 92–93, 108–9, 112, 158, 191, 195

minimum alveolar concentration (MAC), 121

Mirebalais University Hospital, Haiti, 214–16

moods, resources for managing, 269–70

Moore, Gordon, 171, 173

Moore Foundation, 171, 173

Morandi, Dr. Alessandro, 158, 176

morphine, 8, 57, 116, 131, 135, 210–11, 228

MRI, 24, 31, 91, 108, 109, 112, 158, 199, 200

Mullicane, Kyle (patient), 86, 87–89, 91, 92–94, 201

muscle
ICU stays with damage to, 58, 138, 145, 147, 150, 151, 153, 202–3, 215, 234, 270
Long COVID with weakness in, 190
lungs with, 50
physical therapy to regain use of, 146, 150, 151, 202
PICS with weakness in, 138, 207, 259
sliding filament hypothesis of, 152

narcotics
delirium from withdrawal from, 250
ventilated patients with, 169

narrative medicine, 193–94

National Academy of Medicine, 224–25

National Institute on Aging, 175, 249, 281

necrotizing fasciitis, 156, 177

Needham, Dr. Dale, 138

negative-pressure ventilators, 34, 36

Negovsky, Dr. Vladimir Alexandrovitch, 39

nerves
immobilization with damage to, 58
muscle interaction with, 152
PICS and damage to, 138, 150, 207, 270
polio's impact on, 35

neurocognitive testing, 157, 160, 261

neurogenesis, 201, 272

neurological conditions, 78, 98, 267

New England Journal of Medicine, 66, 126, 171, 175

Nightingale, Florence, 32–33
Nordness, Dr. Mina, 86–87
nurses
  A2F safety bundle and, 173, 174,
    175
  burnout suffered by, 224, 225
  COVID care by, 28, 234–35, 236,
    237–39
  critical care and, 32–33, 39
  delirium detection by, 79, 90
  end-of-life care and, 224–26
  ICU diaries and, 184, 253
  physical therapy, 147, 148, 165
  sedative use in ICU and, 122, 130,
    140–41, 234
  social interactions between patients
    and, 181
  3 Wishes Project and, 225
  workshops on ICU improvements
    with, 167–68, 169, 172
nursing homes, 31, 150, 175
nutrition and diet, 251, 266
nutritionists, 137, 265, 280
Nydahl, Dr. Peter, 163, 166

oath (first do no harm), xi
obesity, 206
occupational therapy, 28, 137, 165,
    173, 186, 189, 203, 247, 261,
    265, 267, 269, 270
Ochsner, Dr. Alton, 2, 33
Odense University Hospital, Denmark,
    134–36, 139–41, 142–43, 147,
    154
Of Mice and Men (Steinbeck), 4
Ofri, Dr. Danielle, 210

Oliver Sacks: His Own Life
    (documentary), 210
O'Neal, Dr. Hollis "Bud," 236
"On the Pulse of Morning" (Angelou),
    4, 42–43
opioids, 55, 131, 256, 257
Oppenheimer, J. Robert, 142
organizational challenges, resources for,
    268–69
Osler, Sir (Dr.) William, 70, 78, 236
Outsiders, The (Hinton), 4

PACS (post-acute COVID syndrome),
    190, 262
pain management, 135, 175, 210, 211,
    212, 252, 255, 256, 257
pain medications, 8, 78, 120, 130,
    168, 250
Paine, Thomas, 75, 170
Pale Horse, Pale Rider (Porter), 45
palliative care, 216–20
Pandharipande, Dr. Pratik, 16, 107–8,
    128–29
paralytics, 54, 78
Partners In Health (PIH), 214, 216
PASC (post-acute sequelae of
    SARS-CoV-2 infection), 190,
    262
Patchett, Ann, 86
Patel, Dr. Mayur, 199
patient outcomes, 10, 30, 49, 97, 101,
    106, 140, 147–48, 151, 171,
    182, 193, 205, 264
PEEP (positive end-expiratory
    pressure), 52–53
peripartum cardiomyopathy, 5–6

Perme, Christiane "Chris," 147–50, 153, 173

Petty, Dr. Thomas, 52–53, 57–58, 73–74

physical remediation, resources for, 270–72

physical therapists
ICU patients and, 136, 139, 146, 147–48, 165, 174, 186
ICU survivors and, 202–3, 265
PICS and, 260, 261

physician-assisted suicide, 162

physicians
compassion in relationship between patients and, 143–44
response to ICU patients' needs by, 99–101
seeing the patient as a whole person by, 69–71

Piano, Dr. Giancarlo (patient), 229–31

PICS. *See* post-intensive care syndrome

Pierre Curie (Curie), 27

Pisani, Dr. Margaret, 183

Plan-Do-Study-Act (PDSA) cycles, 170

pneumonia, 8, 19, 21, 28, 52, 75, 128, 149, 150, 185, 209, 213, 214, 230, 244

polio epidemics, ventilator innovation during, 34–37, 50, 133

Porter, Katherine Anne, 45

Portnoy, Dr. Darin, 2, 65, 236–37

positive end-expiratory pressure (PEEP), 52–53

post-acute COVID syndrome, 190, 262

post-acute sequelae of SARS-CoV-2 infection, 190, 262

post-intensive care syndrome (PICS)
brain and body problems after discharge from ICU and, 14–15
caregivers and, 262
cognitive and mental health remediation after, 267–70
COVID-19 and risk for, 262–63
general guide to, 258–62
incidence among ICU survivors, 16
multifold cognitive rehabilitation approach to, 198
patients at risk for, 259–60
range of conditions seen in, 15–16
resources for, 258–67
support groups for, 261, 266, 270
survivor's guide for, 263–67
symptoms of, 258–59

post-traumatic stress disorder (PTSD)
caregivers' risk for, 262
family members of ICU survivors with, 25, 187
ICU diaries and reduction in, 184
ICU survivors with, 24, 90, 92, 160
PICS and, 16, 138, 259
treatment for, 201, 261

Principles of Neural Science (Kandel and Schwartz), 83, 97

Prine, Fiona Whelan, 185

Prine, John, 111, 185

prison, prisoner, imprisoned, 22, 59, 105, 156, 204, 220, 239

prognosis, 115, 217

protocols, 81, 93, 118, 122, 133, 136, 137, 168, 175, 183, 235, 236

Index

PTSD. *See* post-traumatic stress disorder

pulmonary fibrosis, 61, 115

pulmonologists, 60, 80, 81, 145, 148, 242, 265

Pun, Dr. Brenda, 84, 173

qualitative research, 181

quality of life, 10, 11, 22, 87, 164, 169, 217, 259

quantitative research, 181

Ramsay scale, 121

randomized controlled trials, 118, 125, 184

rehabilitation

cognitive, 197–99, 201, 203, 267, 270

physical, 151, 166, 186, 190, 192, 207, 228

rehabilitation therapists, 247, 267

religion

Buddhist, 228

Catholic, 229, 230–31

Hindu, 227

Jewish, 227

Muslim, 227

respiratory therapists, 28, 66, 118, 122, 137, 167, 280

Reyes, Fred (patient), 206–7

Rice, Dr. Todd, 165

Richmond Agitation-Sedation Scale (RASS), 121

Riker, Dr. Richard, 121

Riviello, Dr. Elisabeth, 235

Rogers, Everett, 33

Romano, Dr. John, 79–80

Ross, Heidi (patient), 190

Rowan, Dr. Kathy, 32

Rubin, Eileen, 193

Rush University, 199

Russell, John, 59–60

Russo, Anthony (patient), 23–25, 26, 171

Ruthie the Duck Lady (patient), 1–2

Sacks, Dr. Oliver, 103, 142, 210

Safar, Dr. Peter, 39

safety, 105, 151, 167, 255

St. Cyr, Dr. Carlos, 214, 215–16

Saint Thomas hospital, Nashville, 121–22

SATs (spontaneous awakening trials), 168, 255

Saturday Night (Hunter), 240–41

SBTs (spontaneous breathing trials), 66–67, 168, 178, 255

SCCM (Society of Critical Care Medicine), 173–74, 175, 189, 255

Schiro, Elena, 165–66

Schwartz, Dr. James, 83, 97

Schweickert, Dr. Bill, 139, 154

science, 83, 100, 107, 129, 131–32, 141, 142, 168–69, 171, 176, 205–6, 230, 235–36, 242

screening

for ICU delirium, 86, 251, 257

before transplantation, 60–61

"sedate and immobilize" standard of care

criticism of, 57–58

ICU patients' experiences of, 54–56, 130–32

ICU psychosis as side effect in, 56, 79, 112, 131

medical complications in ICU with, 58

sedatives and sedation

anxiety in ICU and, 8, 130, 135, 234

brain monitoring of action of, 126–27

dexmedetomidine trial with, 123–25

early mobility after using, 137–39

intubated patients and, 120

randomized controlled trials of, 118, 122–23, 127–29

Sedation Agitation Scale (SAS), 121

senescence, 21

Separate Peace, A (Knowles), 4

sepsis

delirium risk related to, 250

helpful websites for, 274–75

ICU patients' experiences of, 19, 39, 54, 92, 135, 156, 192, 202, 216

septic shock

ICU death rates over time from, 32

Sessler, Dr. Curt, 121

Sevin, Dr. Carla, 17, 188–89

Shaw, Louis Agassiz Jr., 34

Shem, Samuel, 69

shock, 5, 8, 23, 78, 182, 189, 223, 243, 245

shortness of breath, 41, 61, 190, 210, 238, 258, 270

Skrobik, Dr. Yoanna, 86

sleep problems, 9, 24, 79, 83, 182–83, 249, 256, 259

sleep promotion, 251, 252, 254, 266, 271, 273

sleep protocols, 93, 183, 185

Smith, Dr. Heidi, 186

social determinants of health, 205

Society of Critical Care Medicine (SCCM), 173–74, 175, 189, 255

Solnit, Rebecca, 142

spiritual advisers, 247, 264

Spiritual Exercises (Ignatius of Loyola), 69

spiritual gestures and conversations, in healing, 143

spiritual health, 217, 221

spiritual history, 227, 230

spirituality of patients, 83

end-of-life care and, 227–29, 230–31

isolation and, 105

spiritual needs of patients, 105, 194, 211, 228

spontaneous awakening trials (SATs), 168, 255

spontaneous breathing trials (SBTs), 66–67, 168, 178, 255

Sprung, Dr. Charlie, 217

Spuhler, Vicki, 168

State of Wonder (Patchett), 86

statistics, 164

Steinbeck, John, 4, 137, 150–51

Stevens, Doyle Thomas "DT" and Virginia (patients), 237–38

story, power of, in ICU survivors' support groups, 193–94

stroke, 66, 157, 197, 198, 199

Strøm, Dr. Thomas, 134–36, 137, 140–41, 148, 154

subcutaneous emphysema, 29–30

suicide

burnout in doctors and nurses and, 224

after ICU stay, 7–8, 159

physician-assisted, 162

possible reasons behind, 161–62

Sundloff, Joy (patient), 144–47, 153, 215

support groups for ICU survivors

CIBS' organizing of, 16–17, 86, 247

COVID survivors in, 190

delirium stories shared in, 86–94

first recorded meeting of, 193

helpful websites for, 274–75

hospitals' provision of, as form of rehab and recovery, 192–93

ICU survivors' experience of, 17, 191–92

PICS treatment with, 261, 266, 270

Vanderbilt ICU Recovery Center and, 190, 193

support system

for families of ICU patients, 217

home life for ICU survivors and, 145

ICU survivors' need for, 123, 163, 203

patient-centered and family-centered care in, 217

PICS treatment and, 261, 262

surgeons, tips about delirium for, 257

surgery, 2. *See also* transplantation

communicating feelings to surgeons in, 210

delirium risk related to, 250, 251

first use of general anesthesia in, 120

lung infection after, 14

monitoring brain function during, 126

recovery rooms after, 33

septic shock during, 144

survivorship, 106, 245. *See also* ICU survivors

Sutter Health hospital system, California, 171–72

synapses, 84, 199–200

synaptogenesis, 201

System 1 thinking, 196, 199

System 2 thinking, 196, 198–99

Taub, Dr. Edward, 196, 197–98

taxi drivers, 200

TBI (traumatic brain injury), 157, 199

teamwork, 170

thinking

System 1, 196, 199

System 2, 196, 198–99

Thinking, Fast and Slow (Kahneman), 196

This Side of Paradise (Fitzgerald), 65–66

3 Wishes Project, 218–19

THRIVE Initiative, Society of Critical Care Medicine, 189

Tipping Point, The (Gladwell), 168

Tobin, Dr. Martin, 66

Toft, Dr. Palle, 134, 139–40, 141

toxic shock syndrome, 156
tracheotomies, in polio care, 36–37
transplantation, lung and heart-lung,
    58–62, 65
  decision to move into, 58–59
  first lung transplant surgery in,
    59–60
  monitoring of patient after, 68–69
  patients' experiences of, 63–65,
    67–69, 71, 72–73
  physician's knowledge of patients'
    stories in, 61–62
  screening before, 60–61
  seeing the patient as a whole person
    in, 69–71
trauma, 1, 3, 4, 49, 92, 96–97, 192,
    202, 222
traumatic brain injury (TBI), 157,
    199
Trulock, Dr. Bert, 60–61, 62, 67
Trzeciak, Dr. Stephen, 226
Tulane Medical School, 2, 51, 59, 70,
    196

unconsciousness, medically induced,
    xi, 118, 119–20, 121, 126
unconscious patients, 7, 8, 19, 56, 57,
    117, 119, 123, 135
University Hospital of Mirebalais,
    Haiti, 214–16
upstream problems, 205, 206

vaccines, 185
Vanderbilt University Medical Center,
    Nashville
  CIBS Center at. See CIBS Center

ICU Recovery Center at, 188–89,
    190, 193
ventilators
  COVID patients and, 28
  innovation during polio epidemics
    in, 34–37, 50, 133
  intense sedation and paralysis used
    with, 53–56
  inverse ratio ventilation (IRV)
    readings in, 53–54
  negative-pressure approach to, 34, 36
  positive end-expiratory pressure
    (PEEP) readings with, 52–53
  spontaneous breathing trials (SBTs)
    with, 66–67, 168, 178
Verghese, Dr. Abraham, 115, 225
veterans, as patients, 228
Veterans Affairs, Department of, 110,
    198
Veterans Affairs Hospital, Nashville,
    174, 204, 209
Vincent, Dr. Jean-Louis, 32
VISIONS program, 158

Wake Forest Medical Center, Winston-
    Salem, North Carolina, 40, 62,
    65, 68, 80, 207
Wald, Dr. Hedy, 194
weakness, resources for, 270–71
weaning standards, for ventilators,
    66–67
Webb, Dr. Watts, 51, 59
Wechsler Adult Intelligence Scale
    (WAIS), 20–21
"Weighing, The" (Hirshfield),
    209

Weil, Dr. Max Harry, 39
well-being, 129, 200, 203, 222
wellness, 217, 274
West, Danny (patient), 72–73
Wheeler, Dr. Art, 165, 164
When Breath Becomes Air (Kalanithi),
   13
White, Dr. Doug, 217
Whitman, Walt, 233

Wilson, Dr. Philip, 221
Wright, Wilbur, 155

Young Men and Fire (Maclean), 1,
   166–67

Zanmi Lasante (ZL), 214
Zitter, Dr. Jessica, 217
Zulman, Dr. Donna, 225

About the Author

E. Wesley Ely, MD, MPH, is an internist, pulmonologist, and critical care physician. Dr. Ely earned his MD at Tulane University School of Medicine, in conjunction with a master's in public health. He serves as the Grant W. Liddle endowed chair in medicine and is a physician-scientist and tenured professor at Vanderbilt University Medical Center. He is also the associate director of aging research for the Tennessee Valley Veteran's Affairs Geriatric Research Education Clinical Center (GRECC). Dr. Ely has had studies published in the *New England Journal of Medicine*, *JAMA*, and *The Lancet*, and his writing has appeared in the *Wall Street Journal*, the *Washington Post*, *USA Today*, and numerous other publications. He lives in Nashville and is the founder and codirector of the Critical Illness, Brain Dysfunction, and Survivorship (CIBS) Center, an organization devoted to research and ongoing care for people affected by critical illness. Dr. Ely is donating all his net proceeds from this book to a fund at the CIBS Center established to help ICU survivors and their families. Visit www.icudelirium.org.